This journal belongs to

_____

Due Date

_____

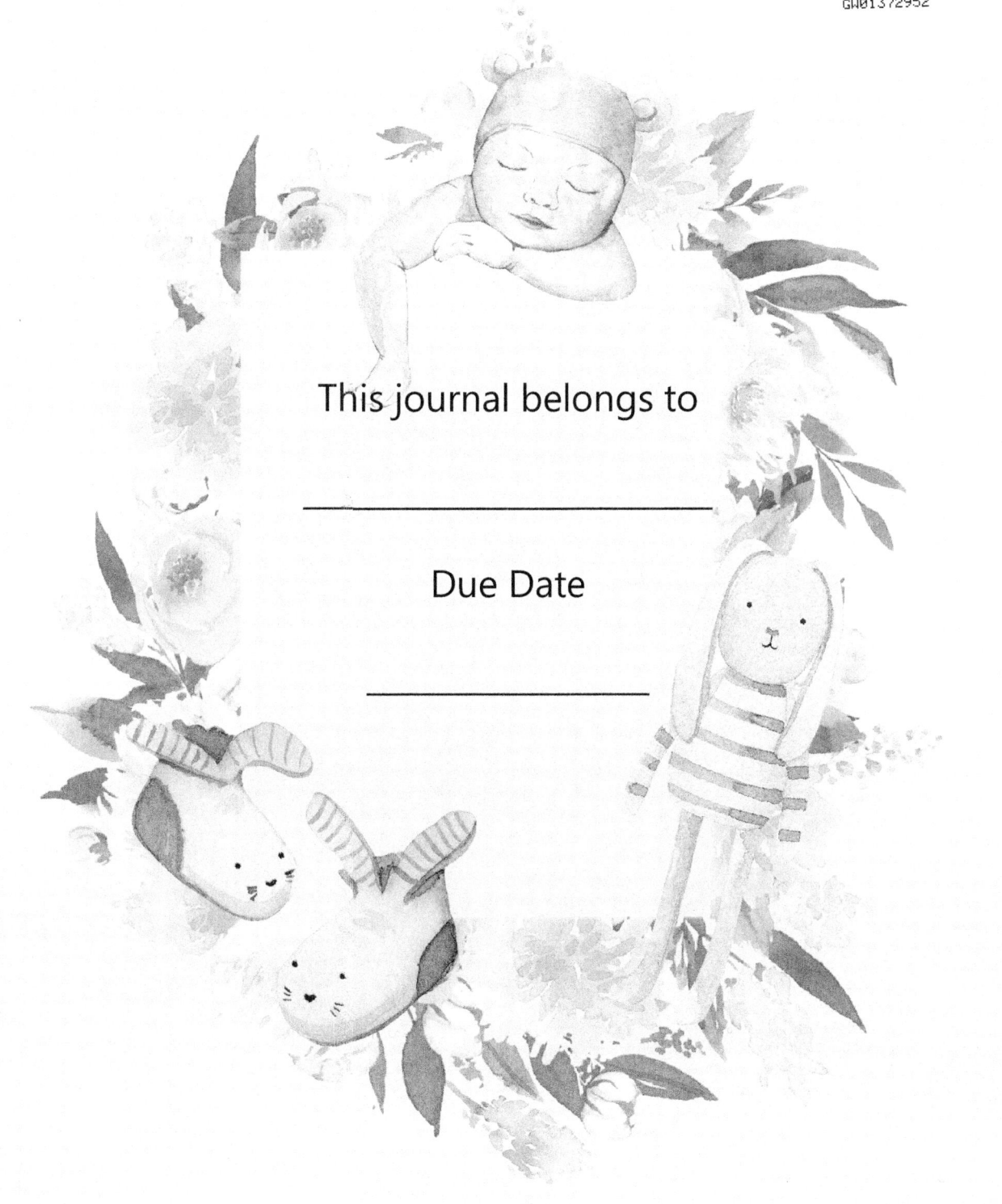

© 2020
William Ralph

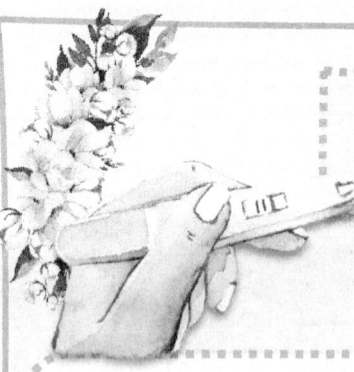

"Dear Baby"

I'm expecting you!

How I suspected I was pregnant

How I felt when I found out

How I told your father

How your father reacted

How we told your siblings and grandparents

How we announced to the world

Our nicknames for you

My special note to you, as we start this journey together

Love, Mom

Pregnancy Planning

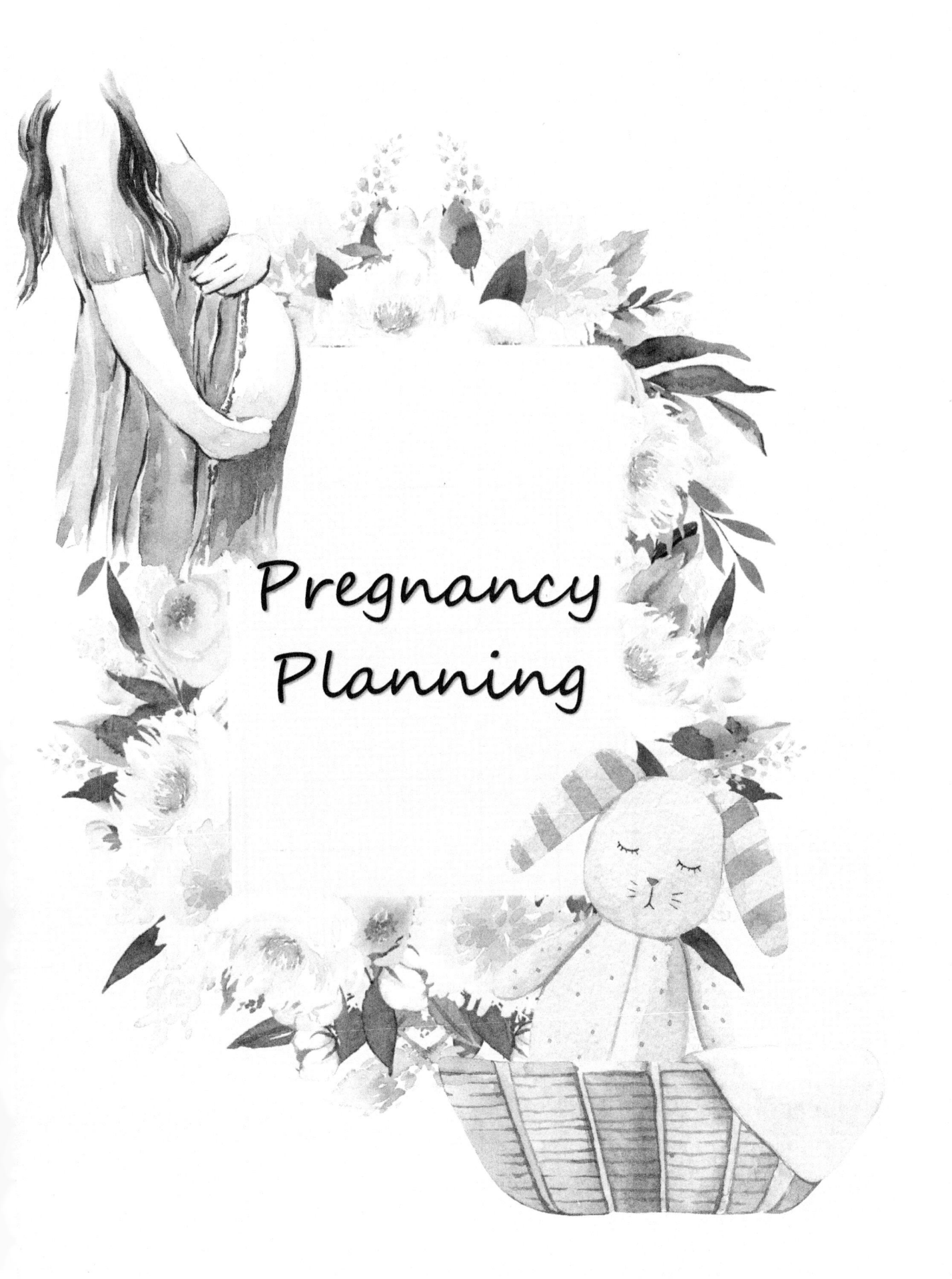

Month							
Week	Mon	Tue	Wed	Thu	Fri	Sat	Sun
	—	—	—	—	—	—	—
	—	—	—	—	—	—	—
	—	—	—	—	—	—	—
	—	—	—	—	—	—	—
	—	—	—	—	—	—	—
	—	—	—	—	—	—	—

Month							
Week	Mon	Tue	Wed	Thu	Fri	Sat	Sun
	—	—	—	—	—	—	—
	—	—	—	—	—	—	—
	—	—	—	—	—	—	—
	—	—	—	—	—	—	—
	—	—	—	—	—	—	—
	—	—	—	—	—	—	—

Notes

Month

Week	Mon	Tue	Wed	Thu	Fri	Sat	Sun
	—	—	—	—	—	—	—
	—	—	—	—	—	—	—
	—	—	—	—	—	—	—
	—	—	—	—	—	—	—
	—	—	—	—	—	—	—
	—	—	—	—	—	—	—

Notes

Month

Week	Mon	Tue	Wed	Thu	Fri	Sat	Sun
	—	—	—	—	—	—	—
	—	—	—	—	—	—	—
	—	—	—	—	—	—	—
	—	—	—	—	—	—	—
	—	—	—	—	—	—	—
	—	—	—	—	—	—	—

Month							
Week	Mon	Tue	Wed	Thu	Fri	Sat	Sun
	—	—	—	—	—	—	—
	—	—	—	—	—	—	—
	—	—	—	—	—	—	—
	—	—	—	—	—	—	—
	—	—	—	—	—	—	—
	—	—	—	—	—	—	—

Notes

Month							
Week	Mon	Tue	Wed	Thu	Fri	Sat	Sun
	—	—	—	—	—	—	—
	—	—	—	—	—	—	—
	—	—	—	—	—	—	—
	—	—	—	—	—	—	—
	—	—	—	—	—	—	—
	—	—	—	—	—	—	—

Month

Week	Mon	Tue	Wed	Thu	Fri	Sat	Sun
	—	—	—	—	—	—	—
	—	—	—	—	—	—	—
	—	—	—	—	—	—	—
	—	—	—	—	—	—	—
	—	—	—	—	—	—	—
	—	—	—	—	—	—	—

Month

Week	Mon	Tue	Wed	Thu	Fri	Sat	Sun
	—	—	—	—	—	—	—
	—	—	—	—	—	—	—
	—	—	—	—	—	—	—
	—	—	—	—	—	—	—
	—	—	—	—	—	—	—
	—	—	—	—	—	—	—

Notes

Weekly To Do List

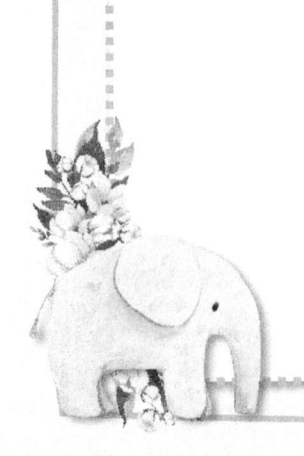

Week _____

Monday
- ○ ------------------
- ○ ------------------
- ○ ------------------
- ○ ------------------
- ○ ------------------

Appointments
___ / ___ ------------
___ / ___ ------------

Tuesday
- ○ ------------------
- ○ ------------------
- ○ ------------------
- ○ ------------------
- ○ ------------------

Appointments
___ / ___ ------------
___ / ___ ------------

Wednesday
- ○ ------------------
- ○ ------------------
- ○ ------------------
- ○ ------------------
- ○ ------------------

Appointments
___ / ___ ------------
___ / ___ ------------

Thursday
- ○ ------------------
- ○ ------------------
- ○ ------------------
- ○ ------------------
- ○ ------------------

Appointments
___ / ___ ------------
___ / ___ ------------

Friday
- ○ ------------------
- ○ ------------------
- ○ ------------------
- ○ ------------------
- ○ ------------------

Appointments
___ / ___ ------------
___ / ___ ------------

Saturday
- ○ ------------------
- ○ ------------------
- ○ ------------------
- ○ ------------------
- ○ ------------------
- ○ ------------------
- ○ ------------------

Sunday
- ○ ------------------
- ○ ------------------
- ○ ------------------
- ○ ------------------
- ○ ------------------
- ○ ------------------
- ○ ------------------

Weekly To Do List

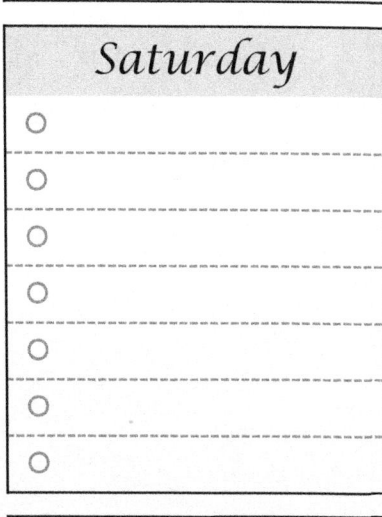

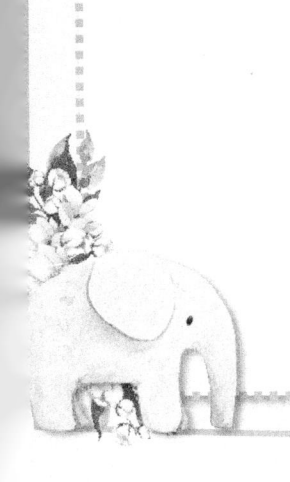

Week _____

Monday
- ○ _____
- ○ _____
- ○ _____
- ○ _____
- ○ _____

Appointments
___/___
___/___

Tuesday
- ○ _____
- ○ _____
- ○ _____
- ○ _____
- ○ _____

Appointments
___/___
___/___

Wednesday
- ○ _____
- ○ _____
- ○ _____
- ○ _____
- ○ _____

Appointments
___/___
___/___

Thursday
- ○ _____
- ○ _____
- ○ _____
- ○ _____
- ○ _____

Appointments
___/___
___/___

Friday
- ○ _____
- ○ _____
- ○ _____
- ○ _____
- ○ _____

Appointments
___/___
___/___

Saturday
- ○ _____
- ○ _____
- ○ _____
- ○ _____
- ○ _____
- ○ _____
- ○ _____

Sunday
- ○ _____
- ○ _____
- ○ _____
- ○ _____
- ○ _____
- ○ _____
- ○ _____

Weekly To Do List

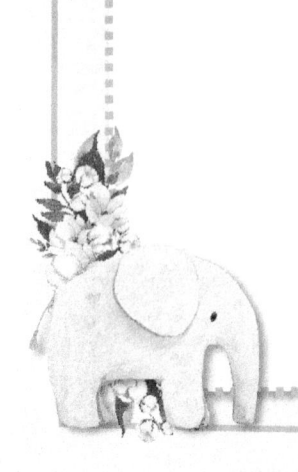

Week _____

Monday
- ○ _____
- ○ _____
- ○ _____
- ○ _____
- ○ _____

Appointments
____ / ____
____ / ____

Tuesday
- ○ _____
- ○ _____
- ○ _____
- ○ _____
- ○ _____

Appointments
____ / ____
____ / ____

Wednesday
- ○ _____
- ○ _____
- ○ _____
- ○ _____
- ○ _____

Appointments
____ / ____
____ / ____

Thursday
- ○ _____
- ○ _____
- ○ _____
- ○ _____
- ○ _____

Appointments
____ / ____
____ / ____

Friday
- ○ _____
- ○ _____
- ○ _____
- ○ _____
- ○ _____

Appointments
____ / ____
____ / ____

Saturday
- ○ _____
- ○ _____
- ○ _____
- ○ _____
- ○ _____
- ○ _____
- ○ _____

Sunday
- ○ _____
- ○ _____
- ○ _____
- ○ _____
- ○ _____
- ○ _____
- ○ _____

Weekly To Do List

Week _____

Monday
- ○ ----------------
- ○ ----------------
- ○ ----------------
- ○ ----------------
- ○ ----------------

Appointments
___ / ___
___ / ___

Tuesday
- ○ ----------------
- ○ ----------------
- ○ ----------------
- ○ ----------------
- ○ ----------------

Appointments
___ / ___
___ / ___

Wednesday
- ○ ----------------
- ○ ----------------
- ○ ----------------
- ○ ----------------
- ○ ----------------

Appointments
___ / ___
___ / ___

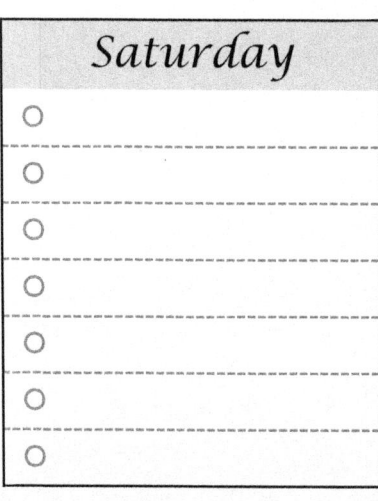

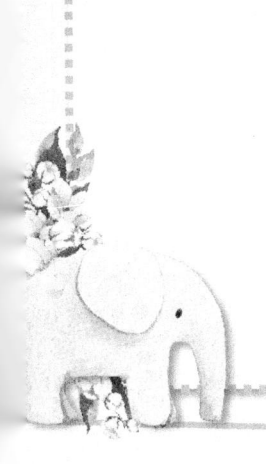

Thursday
- ○ ----------------
- ○ ----------------
- ○ ----------------
- ○ ----------------
- ○ ----------------

Appointments
___ / ___
___ / ___

Friday
- ○ ----------------
- ○ ----------------
- ○ ----------------
- ○ ----------------
- ○ ----------------

Appointments
___ / ___
___ / ___

Saturday
- ○ ----------------
- ○ ----------------
- ○ ----------------
- ○ ----------------
- ○ ----------------
- ○ ----------------
- ○ ----------------

Sunday
- ○ ----------------
- ○ ----------------
- ○ ----------------
- ○ ----------------
- ○ ----------------
- ○ ----------------
- ○ ----------------

Weekly To Do List

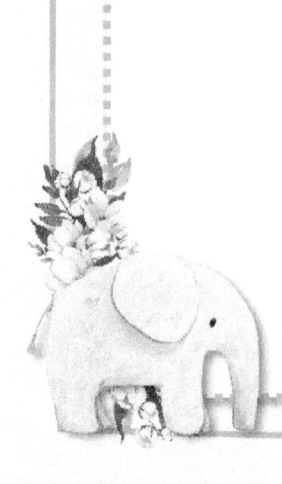

Week _____

Monday
- ○
- ○
- ○
- ○
- ○

Appointments
___ / ___
___ / ___

Tuesday
- ○
- ○
- ○
- ○
- ○

Appointments
___ / ___
___ / ___

Wednesday
- ○
- ○
- ○
- ○
- ○

Appointments
___ / ___
___ / ___

Thursday
- ○
- ○
- ○
- ○
- ○

Appointments
___ / ___
___ / ___

Friday
- ○
- ○
- ○
- ○
- ○

Appointments
___ / ___
___ / ___

Saturday
- ○
- ○
- ○
- ○
- ○
- ○
- ○

Sunday
- ○
- ○
- ○
- ○
- ○
- ○
- ○

Weekly To Do List

Week _____

Monday
- ○ _____
- ○ _____
- ○ _____
- ○ _____
- ○ _____

Appointments
___ / ___
___ / ___

Tuesday
- ○ _____
- ○ _____
- ○ _____
- ○ _____
- ○ _____

Appointments
___ / ___
___ / ___

Wednesday
- ○ _____
- ○ _____
- ○ _____
- ○ _____
- ○ _____

Appointments
___ / ___
___ / ___

Thursday
- ○ _____
- ○ _____
- ○ _____
- ○ _____
- ○ _____

Appointments
___ / ___
___ / ___

Friday
- ○ _____
- ○ _____
- ○ _____
- ○ _____
- ○ _____

Appointments
___ / ___
___ / ___

Saturday
- ○ _____
- ○ _____
- ○ _____
- ○ _____
- ○ _____
- ○ _____
- ○ _____

Sunday
- ○ _____
- ○ _____
- ○ _____
- ○ _____
- ○ _____
- ○ _____
- ○ _____

Weekly To Do List

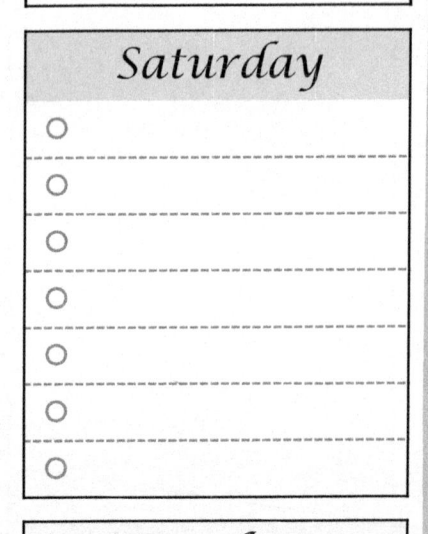

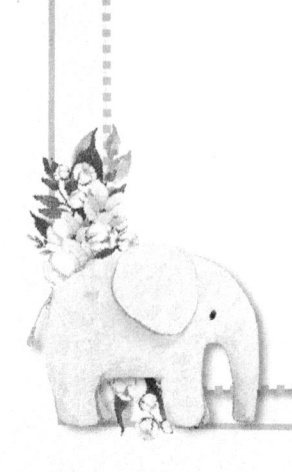

Week _____

Monday
- ○ ─────────
- ○ ─────────
- ○ ─────────
- ○ ─────────
- ○ ─────────

Appointments
___ / ___
___ / ___

Tuesday
- ○ ─────────
- ○ ─────────
- ○ ─────────
- ○ ─────────
- ○ ─────────

Appointments
___ / ___
___ / ___

Wednesday
- ○ ─────────
- ○ ─────────
- ○ ─────────
- ○ ─────────
- ○ ─────────

Appointments
___ / ___
___ / ___

Thursday
- ○ ─────────
- ○ ─────────
- ○ ─────────
- ○ ─────────
- ○ ─────────

Appointments
___ / ___
___ / ___

Friday
- ○ ─────────
- ○ ─────────
- ○ ─────────
- ○ ─────────
- ○ ─────────

Appointments
___ / ___
___ / ___

Saturday
- ○ ─────────
- ○ ─────────
- ○ ─────────
- ○ ─────────
- ○ ─────────
- ○ ─────────
- ○ ─────────

Sunday
- ○ ─────────
- ○ ─────────
- ○ ─────────
- ○ ─────────
- ○ ─────────
- ○ ─────────
- ○ ─────────

Important Contacts

Emergency	Who		Contact No.	

Gynecologist	Name			
Contact No.	Email	Address	Notes	

Midwife	Name			
Contact No.	Email	Address	Notes	

Partner	Name			
Contact No.	Email	Address	Notes	

Hospital	Name			
Contact No.	Email	Address	Notes	

	Name			
Contact No.	Email	Address	Notes	

Prenatal Appointments

Date	Time	Doctor		
Questions for Doctor			**My weight**	
			My BP	
Baby Stats						
Gestation Age	Heartbeat	Length	Head	Abdomen	Femur

Notes

Date	Time	Doctor		
Questions for Doctor			**My weight**	
			My BP	
Baby Stats						
Gestation Age	Heartbeat	Length	Head	Abdomen	Femur

Notes

Antenatal Classes

Where		When	
Instructor		Tel	
Start Date		Cost	
Postnatal support	____ Yes ____ No		

Attendance Log

Date	Topic
Notes	
Questions for next session	

Date	Topic
Notes	
Questions for next session	

Date	Topic
Notes	
Questions for next session	

Date	Topic
Notes	
Questions for next session	

Date	Topic
Notes	
Questions for next session	

Date	Topic
Notes	
Questions for next session	

Antenatal Classes Attendance Log

Date	Topic

Notes

Questions for next session

Date	Topic

Notes

Questions for next session

Date	Topic

Notes

Questions for next session

Date	Topic

Notes

Questions for next session

Date	Topic

Notes

Questions for next session

Date	Topic

Notes

Questions for next session

Date	Topic

Notes

Questions for next session

Date	Topic

Notes

Questions for next session

Resources

Resource	Person	Book	Website	Movie	Other	Where to find	Notes

Healthy Eating

Healthy Foods for Baby and Me	Foods to Avoid

Weekly Meal Planner

Week _____

	Vitamins & Water	Breakfast	Lunch	Dinner	Snacks	Notes
Monday						
Tuesday						
Wednesday						
Thursday						
Friday						
Saturday						
Sunday						

Weekly Meal Planner

Week _____

	Vitamins & Water	Breakfast	Lunch	Dinner	Snacks	Notes
Monday						
Tuesday						
Wednesday						
Thursday						
Friday						
Saturday						
Sunday						

Weekly Meal Planner

Week _____

	Vitamins & Water	Breakfast	Lunch	Dinner	Snacks	Notes
Monday						
Tuesday						
Wednesday						
Thursday						
Friday						
Saturday						
Sunday						

Weekly Meal Planner

Week _____

	Vitamins & Water	Breakfast	Lunch	Dinner	Snacks	Notes
Monday						
Tuesday						
Wednesday						
Thursday						
Friday						
Saturday						
Sunday						

Weekly Meal Planner

Week _____

	Vitamins & Water	Breakfast	Lunch	Dinner	Snacks	Notes
Monday						
Tuesday						
Wednesday						
Thursday						
Friday						
Saturday						
Sunday						

Weekly Meal Planner

Week _____

	Vitamins & Water	Breakfast	Lunch	Dinner	Snacks	Notes
Monday						
Tuesday						
Wednesday						
Thursday						
Friday						
Saturday						
Sunday						

Weekly Meal Planner

Week _____

	Vitamins & Water	Breakfast	Lunch	Dinner	Snacks	Notes
Monday						
Tuesday						
Wednesday						
Thursday						
Friday						
Saturday						
Sunday						

Weekly Meal Planner

Week _____

	Vitamins & Water	Breakfast	Lunch	Dinner	Snacks	Notes
Monday						
Tuesday						
Wednesday						
Thursday						
Friday						
Saturday						
Sunday						

Frozen Meals

Meal	Date Prepared	Number of Servings	Notes

Doula Questionnaire

Name:	Email:	Tel:

What kind of training do you have? When and where did you qualify?	
Do you participate in continuing education?	
Why did you become a doula?	
Describe your doula style.	
How many births have you attended?	
Will you be available on and around my due date?	
What are your fees and what's included? Do you have different package offerings?	
Have you given birth yourself?	
Do you have any other clients with due dates close to mine?	
Do you have a backup doula? When will you introduce her?	
Do you make visits before and after the birth?	
Are you available for me to contact you any time with questions or concerns?	
What is your experience with birth complications?	
Have you attended home births?	
Have you attended births that ended up as c-sections?	
Is there a time limit to your birth attendance? What do you do in the case of long labor?	
How do you work with my doctor, midwife, partner?	
What is your approach to me while I'm in labor?	
What is your opinion on pain medications and epidurals?	
How long do you stay after the birth?	
What do you believe are the best coping techniques?	
Where can I get references / reviews from previous clients?	
What additional services do you offer? What are the fees?	

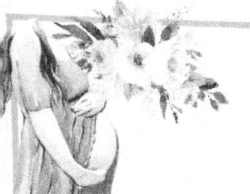

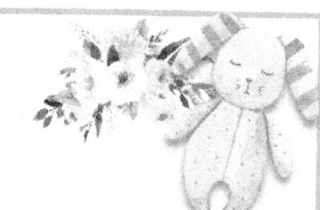

Birthing Plan

Hospital		Contact No.		Notes
Medical Insurance	Policy	Policy Number	Contact No.	
Prenatal Visit	Date/Time	Contact Person		

Prenatal Visit Questions / Notes

Due Date		Induction Date	
My Full Name			
Partner's Full Name			
Doctor		Contact No.	
Midwife		Contact No.	

Preferred Birthing Plan

○ Natural ○ Caesarean ○ Water Birth ○ VBAC ○ Other

Alternate Choice	
Important Information	Blood Group
	Allergies
	Other

Hospital Packing List

for Baby

- ○ _____
- ○ _____
- ○ _____
- ○ _____
- ○ _____
- ○ _____

- ○ _____
- ○ _____
- ○ _____
- ○ _____
- ○ _____
- ○ _____

Have ready by
Date:

for Mom

- ○ _____
- ○ _____
- ○ _____
- ○ _____
- ○ _____
- ○ _____

- ○ _____
- ○ _____
- ○ _____
- ○ _____
- ○ _____
- ○ _____

Notes

_____
_____
_____
_____
_____

for Partner

- ○ _____
- ○ _____
- ○ _____
- ○ _____
- ○ _____
- ○ _____

- ○ _____
- ○ _____
- ○ _____
- ○ _____
- ○ _____
- ○ _____

_____
_____
_____
_____
_____
_____

Partner's Checklist

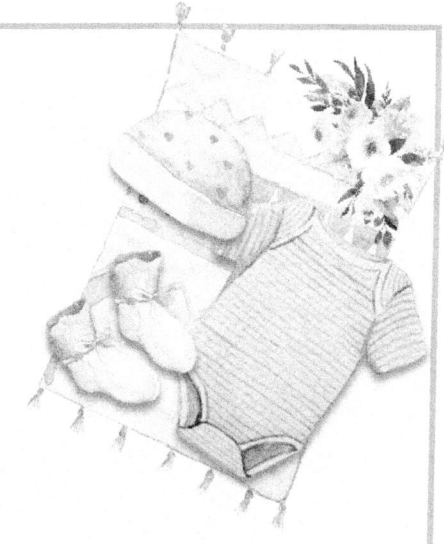

To Do	Done
Arrange child minders for older children	○
Gifts for Mom and Baby	○
Notify people on Contact List	○
Register Baby	○
Household management and meals:	
	○
	○
	○
	○
	○
	○
	○
	○
Other:	
	○
	○
	○
	○
	○
	○
	○
	○
	○
	○
	○
	○

Notes

People to Notify

Notes

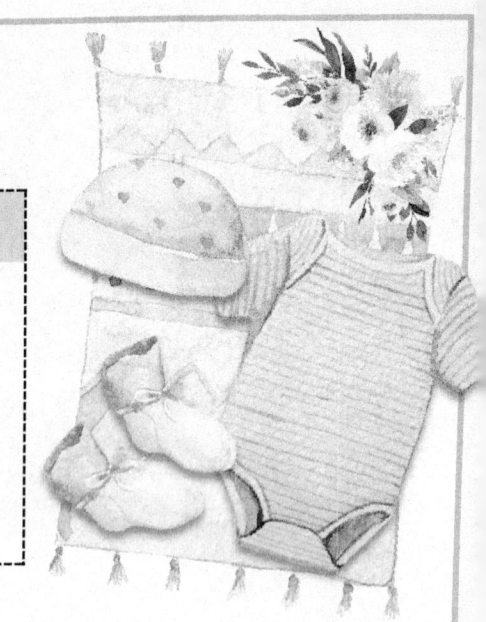

Name	Contact No.	Email	Done	Notes
			○	
			○	
			○	
			○	
			○	
			○	
			○	
			○	
			○	
			○	
			○	
			○	
			○	
			○	
			○	
			○	
			○	

Postnatal Planning

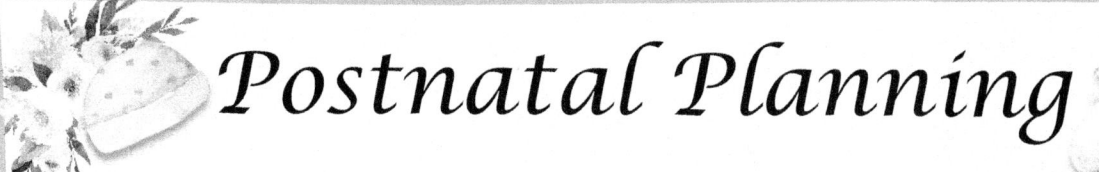

Will I be a stay at home mom, or will I return to work after maternity leave?	
When to announce pregnancy at work	
When to hand in resignation / book maternity leave	
Plan for income during maternity leave / alternate income as a stay at home mom	
What are my childcare options?	
Final choice for childcare	
Alternative for childcare	

Childcare Options

Name	Contact No.	Email	Notes

Preparing for Baby

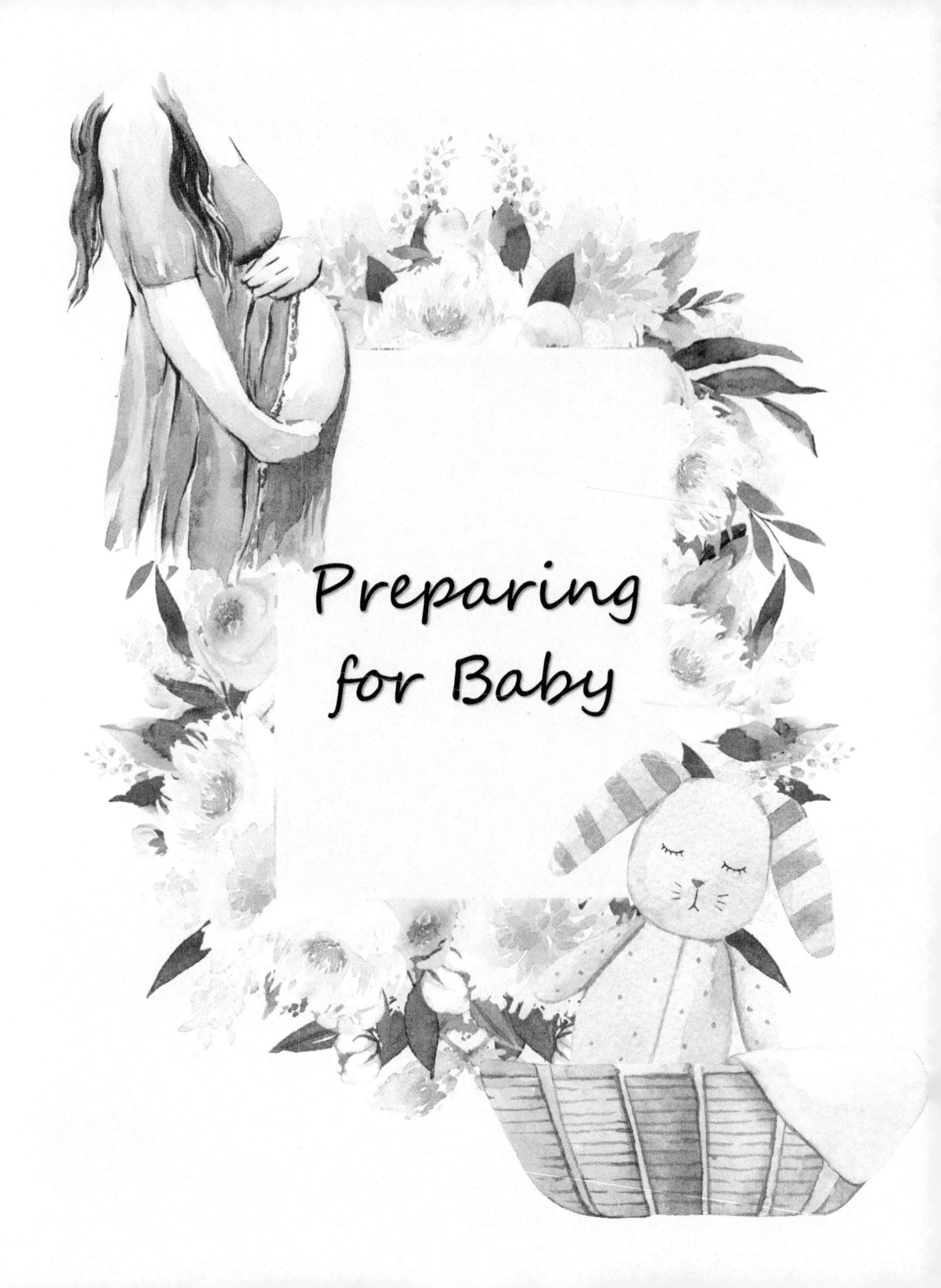

Boys' Names

Names I like	Names my Partner likes

Short List

First Name	Middle Name

Girls' Names

Names I like	Names my Partner likes

Short List

First Name	Middle Name

Baby Budget

Item	Budget	Actual	Date Purchased	Where Purchased
TOTAL				

Notes

Nursery Ideas

Themes

Colors

Furniture

Decor

Nursery Layout

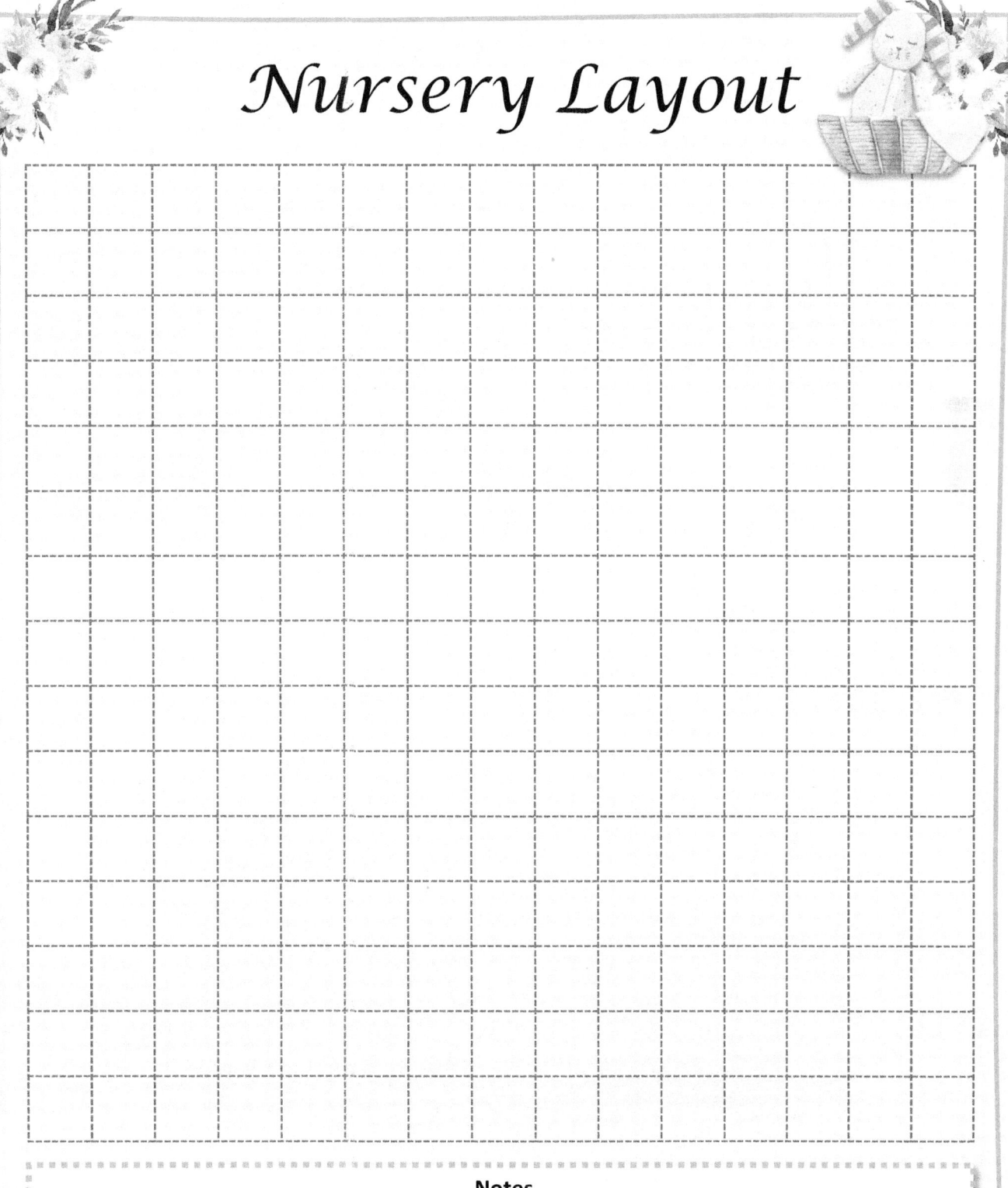

Notes

Nursery Wish List

Item	Source	Cost	Add to Registry?

Nursery Checklist

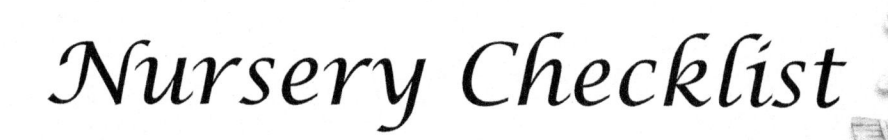

To Do	Done	To Buy	Done
	○		○
	○		○
	○		○
	○		○
	○		○
	○		○
	○		○
	○		○
	○		○
	○		○
	○		○
	○		○
	○		○
	○		○
	○		○
	○		○
	○		○
	○		○
	○		○
	○		○
	○		○
	○		○
	○		○
	○		○
	○		○
	○		○

Baby-Proofing the Home

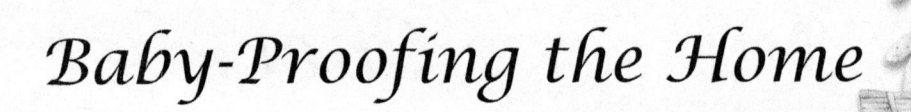

To Do	Done	To Buy	Done
Check and cover sharp edges	○	Plug socket covers	○
Hide all loose cables	○	Baby Gates for Staircase & doorways	○
Medicines in high cupboard	○	Fireplace Screen	○
Cleaning chemicals in high cupboard	○	Cupboard Latches	○
Check First Aid Kit	○		○
Emergency numbers list	○		○
Non-slip pads under rugs	○		○
Poisonous plants removed	○		○

Baby Shower Registry

Where registered

Item	Qty	Details	Received ✓

Baby Shower Memories

Hosted by

Date

Theme

I helped ○   It was a surprise ○

Food and Décor

Games and Activities

Special Memories

Baby Shower Guest & Gift List

Name	Gift	Thank You sent

Pregnancy Trackers

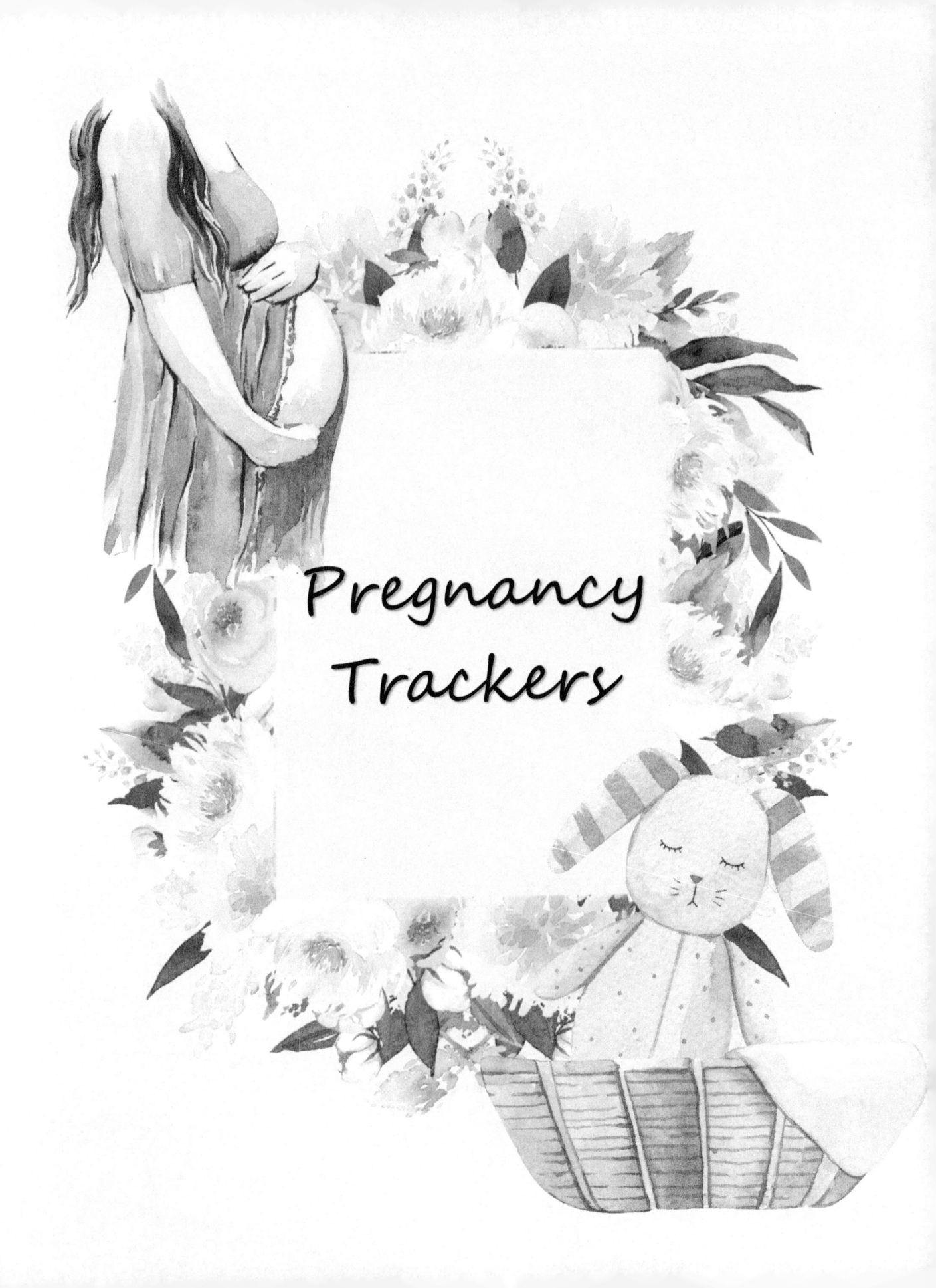

Symptoms Tracker

Date	Time	Food or Activity	Symptoms	Mild	Moderate	Severe	What helped / Notes
				○	○	○	
				○	○	○	
				○	○	○	
				○	○	○	
				○	○	○	
				○	○	○	
				○	○	○	
				○	○	○	
				○	○	○	
				○	○	○	

Weight Log

Week	Weight	Belly Size	Good	Average	Bad	Notes
1			○	○	○	
2			○	○	○	
3			○	○	○	
4			○	○	○	
5			○	○	○	
6			○	○	○	
7			○	○	○	
8			○	○	○	
9			○	○	○	
10			○	○	○	
11			○	○	○	
12			○	○	○	
13			○	○	○	
14			○	○	○	
15			○	○	○	
16			○	○	○	
17			○	○	○	
18			○	○	○	
19			○	○	○	
20			○	○	○	

Week	Weight	Belly Size	Good	Average	Bad	Notes
21			○	○	○	
22			○	○	○	
23			○	○	○	
24			○	○	○	
25			○	○	○	
26			○	○	○	
27			○	○	○	
28			○	○	○	
29			○	○	○	
30			○	○	○	
31			○	○	○	
32			○	○	○	
33			○	○	○	
34			○	○	○	
35			○	○	○	
36			○	○	○	
37			○	○	○	
38			○	○	○	
39			○	○	○	
40			○	○	○	

Belly Pics

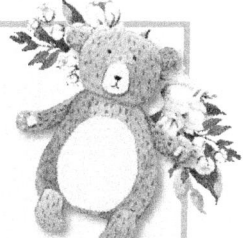

Date

Notes

Date

Notes

Weekly Diet & Exercise Log   **Week** _____

Monday
Vitamins & Water	Breakfast	Lunch	Dinner	Snacks

Exercise:

Notes:

Tuesday
Vitamins & Water	Breakfast	Lunch	Dinner	Snacks

Exercise:

Notes:

Wednesday
Vitamins & Water	Breakfast	Lunch	Dinner	Snacks

Exercise:

Notes:

Thursday
Vitamins & Water	Breakfast	Lunch	Dinner	Snacks

Exercise:

Notes:

Friday
Vitamins & Water	Breakfast	Lunch	Dinner	Snacks

Exercise:

Notes:

Saturday
Vitamins & Water	Breakfast	Lunch	Dinner	Snacks

Exercise:

Notes:

Sunday
Vitamins & Water	Breakfast	Lunch	Dinner	Snacks

Exercise:

Notes:

Weekly Diet & Exercise Log

Week _____

Monday

Vitamins & Water	Breakfast	Lunch	Dinner	Snacks

Exercise:

Notes:

Tuesday

Vitamins & Water	Breakfast	Lunch	Dinner	Snacks

Exercise:

Notes:

Wednesday

Vitamins & Water	Breakfast	Lunch	Dinner	Snacks

Exercise:

Notes:

Thursday

Vitamins & Water	Breakfast	Lunch	Dinner	Snacks

Exercise:

Notes:

Friday

Vitamins & Water	Breakfast	Lunch	Dinner	Snacks

Exercise:

Notes:

Saturday

Vitamins & Water	Breakfast	Lunch	Dinner	Snacks

Exercise:

Notes:

Sunday

Vitamins & Water	Breakfast	Lunch	Dinner	Snacks

Exercise:

Notes:

Weekly Diet & Exercise Log

Week _____

	Vitamins & Water	Breakfast	Lunch	Dinner	Snacks
Monday					

Exercise:
Notes:

	Vitamins & Water	Breakfast	Lunch	Dinner	Snacks
Tuesday					

Exercise:
Notes:

	Vitamins & Water	Breakfast	Lunch	Dinner	Snacks
Wednesday					

Exercise:
Notes:

	Vitamins & Water	Breakfast	Lunch	Dinner	Snacks
Thursday					

Exercise:
Notes:

	Vitamins & Water	Breakfast	Lunch	Dinner	Snacks
Friday					

Exercise:
Notes:

	Vitamins & Water	Breakfast	Lunch	Dinner	Snacks
Saturday					

Exercise:
Notes:

	Vitamins & Water	Breakfast	Lunch	Dinner	Snacks
Sunday					

Exercise:
Notes:

Weekly Diet & Exercise Log

Week _____

Monday
Vitamins & Water	Breakfast	Lunch	Dinner	Snacks

Exercise:

Notes:

Tuesday
Vitamins & Water	Breakfast	Lunch	Dinner	Snacks

Exercise:

Notes:

Wednesday
Vitamins & Water	Breakfast	Lunch	Dinner	Snacks

Exercise:

Notes:

Thursday
Vitamins & Water	Breakfast	Lunch	Dinner	Snacks

Exercise:

Notes:

Friday
Vitamins & Water	Breakfast	Lunch	Dinner	Snacks

Exercise:

Notes:

Saturday
Vitamins & Water	Breakfast	Lunch	Dinner	Snacks

Exercise:

Notes:

Sunday
Vitamins & Water	Breakfast	Lunch	Dinner	Snacks

Exercise:

Notes:

Weekly Diet & Exercise Log

Week _____

	Vitamins & Water	Breakfast	Lunch	Dinner	Snacks
Monday					
Exercise					
Notes					

	Vitamins & Water	Breakfast	Lunch	Dinner	Snacks
Tuesday					
Exercise					
Notes					

	Vitamins & Water	Breakfast	Lunch	Dinner	Snacks
Wednesday					
Exercise					
Notes					

	Vitamins & Water	Breakfast	Lunch	Dinner	Snacks
Thursday					
Exercise					
Notes					

	Vitamins & Water	Breakfast	Lunch	Dinner	Snacks
Friday					
Exercise					
Notes					

	Vitamins & Water	Breakfast	Lunch	Dinner	Snacks
Saturday					
Exercise					
Notes					

	Vitamins & Water	Breakfast	Lunch	Dinner	Snacks
Sunday					
Exercise					
Notes					

Baby Growth Tracker

Weeks

40
39
38
37
36
35
34
33
32
31
30
29
28
27
26
25
24
23
22
21
20
19
18
17
16
15
14
13
12
11
10
9
8
7
6
5
4
3
2
1
0

0   2kg/   4kg/
           4.5lb   9lb

Size / Weight

Notes

Baby Kick Counter

Week 26	Mon	Tues	Wed	Thurs	Fri	Sat	Sun
Start Time							
Stop Time							
Kicks / Movements							

Week 27	Mon	Tues	Wed	Thurs	Fri	Sat	Sun
Start Time							
Stop Time							
Kicks / Movements							

Week 28	Mon	Tues	Wed	Thurs	Fri	Sat	Sun
Start Time							
Stop Time							
Kicks / Movements							

Week 29	Mon	Tues	Wed	Thurs	Fri	Sat	Sun
Start Time							
Stop Time							
Kicks / Movements							

Week 30	Mon	Tues	Wed	Thurs	Fri	Sat	Sun
Start Time							
Stop Time							
Kicks / Movements							

Baby Kick Counter

Week 31	Mon	Tues	Wed	Thurs	Fri	Sat	Sun
Start Time							
Stop Time							
Kicks / Movements							

Week 32	Mon	Tues	Wed	Thurs	Fri	Sat	Sun
Start Time							
Stop Time							
Kicks / Movements							

Week 33	Mon	Tues	Wed	Thurs	Fri	Sat	Sun
Start Time							
Stop Time							
Kicks / Movements							

Week 34	Mon	Tues	Wed	Thurs	Fri	Sat	Sun
Start Time							
Stop Time							
Kicks / Movements							

Week 35	Mon	Tues	Wed	Thurs	Fri	Sat	Sun
Start Time							
Stop Time							
Kicks / Movements							

Baby Kick Counter

Week 36	Mon	Tues	Wed	Thurs	Fri	Sat	Sun
Start Time							
Stop Time							
Kicks / Movements							

Week 37	Mon	Tues	Wed	Thurs	Fri	Sat	Sun
Start Time							
Stop Time							
Kicks / Movements							

Week 38	Mon	Tues	Wed	Thurs	Fri	Sat	Sun
Start Time							
Stop Time							
Kicks / Movements							

Week 39	Mon	Tues	Wed	Thurs	Fri	Sat	Sun
Start Time							
Stop Time							
Kicks / Movements							

Week 40	Mon	Tues	Wed	Thurs	Fri	Sat	Sun
Start Time							
Stop Time							
Kicks / Movements							

Baby Scans

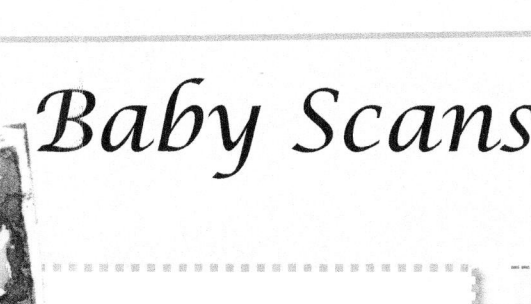

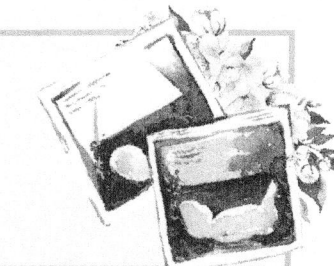

Date

Notes

Date

Notes

First Trimester

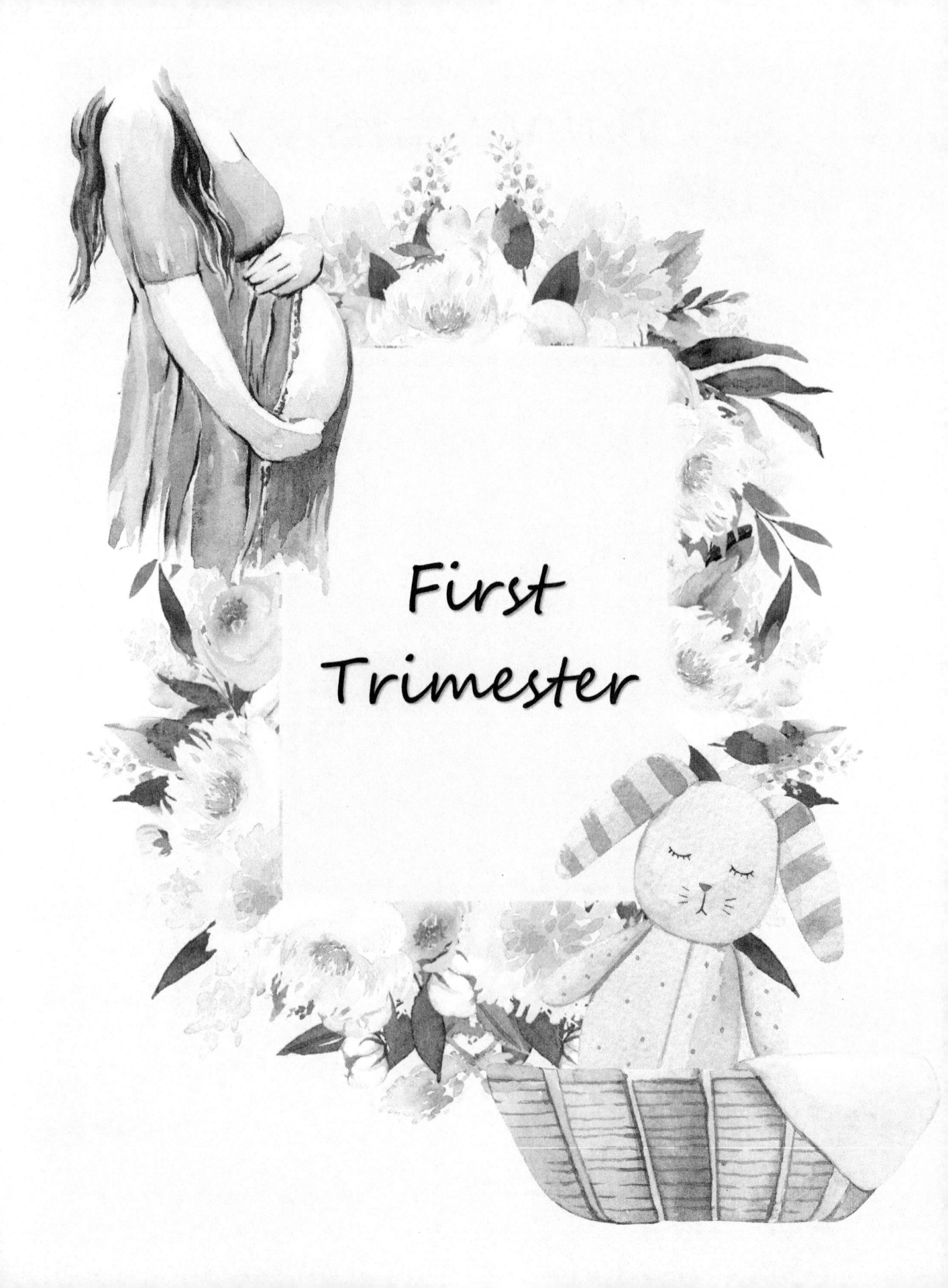

First Trimester

What to Expect

Preparation Checklist

- ○
- ○
- ○
- ○
- ○
- ○
- ○
- ○
- ○
- ○
- ○
- ○
- ○

Notes

I am excited for

I am anxious about

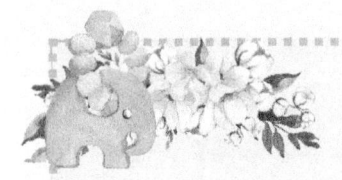

First Trimester Checklist

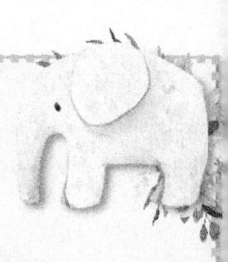

Start taking prenatal vitamin	○
Set up prenatal appointment	○
Manage morning sickness	○
Decide when and how to announce your pregnancy	○
Start practicing healthy eating habits	○
Cut down on caffeine	○
Increase water intake	○
Exercise regularly	○
Research insurance options	○
Be aware of possible complications	○
Start a pregnancy journal and tracker	○
Start taking weekly photos of Baby Bump	○
Start a Baby Budget	○
Get plenty of sleep and rest	○
Don't lift heavy objects	○
Decide whether you're going to hire a doula	○
Research, interview and book your doula	○

Notes

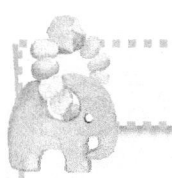

First Trimester

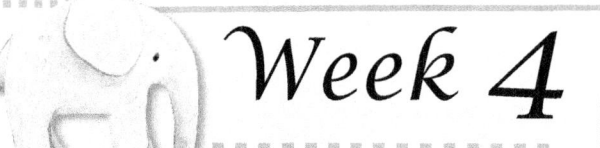

Week 4

Baby's Development

Baby's Weight	
Baby's Size	_____ cm/in
Compares to a...	

About Me

Emotionally I am feeling

My Weight	
My Belly Size	

Events and Appointments

To Do
- ○
- ○
- ○
- ○
- ○
- ○

Cravings

Symptoms

General Health

Special Memories & Notes

"Dear Baby"

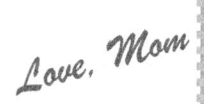

Love, Mom

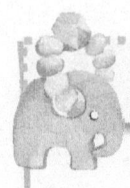

First Trimester

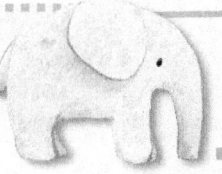

Week 5

Baby's Development

Baby's Weight

Baby's Size _____ cm/in

Compares to a...

About Me

My Weight

Emotionally I am feeling

My Belly Size

Events and Appointments	To Do	
	○	Cravings
	○	
	○	Symptoms
	○	
	○	General Health
	○	

Special Memories & Notes

"Dear Baby"

Love, Mom

First Trimester — Week 6

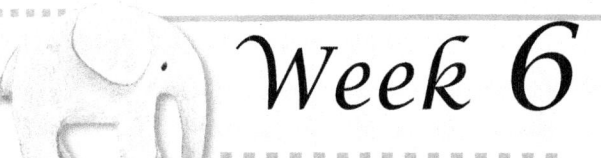

Baby's Development

Baby's Weight	
Baby's Size	_____ cm/in
Compares to a...	

About Me

Emotionally I am feeling

My Weight	
My Belly Size	

Events and Appointments

To Do
- ○
- ○
- ○
- ○
- ○
- ○

Cravings

Symptoms

General Health

Special Memories & Notes

"Dear Baby"

Love, Mom

First Trimester

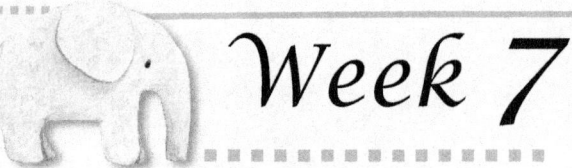

Week 7

Baby's Development

Baby's Weight	
Baby's Size	_____ cm/in
Compares to a...	

About Me
Emotionally I am feeling

My Weight	
My Belly Size	

Events and Appointments	To Do		
	○	Cravings	
	○		
	○	Symptoms	
	○		
	○	General Health	
	○		

Special Memories & Notes

"Dear Baby"

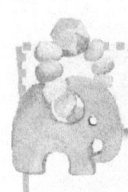

Love, Mom

First Trimester

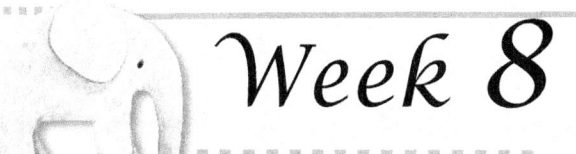

Week 8

Baby's Development

- Baby's Weight
- Baby's Size
- _____ cm/in
- Compares to a...

About Me

Emotionally I am feeling

- My Weight
- My Belly Size

Events and Appointments	To Do	
	○	Cravings
	○	
	○	Symptoms
	○	
	○	General Health
	○	

Special Memories & Notes

"Dear Baby"

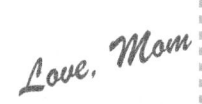

Love, Mom

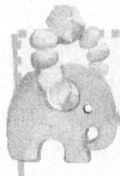

First Trimester

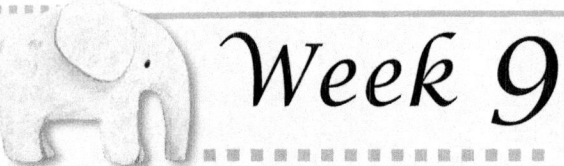

Week 9

Baby's Development

Baby's Weight	
Baby's Size	_____ cm/in
Compares to a...	

About Me

Emotionally I am feeling

My Weight	
My Belly Size	

Events and Appointments	To Do	
	○	Cravings
	○	
	○	Symptoms
	○	
	○	General Health
	○	

Special Memories & Notes

"Dear Baby"

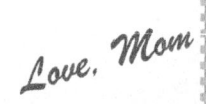

Love, Mom

First Trimester

Week 10

Baby's Development

- Baby's Weight
- Baby's Size _____ cm/in
- Compares to a...

About Me

Emotionally I am feeling

- My Weight
- My Belly Size

Events and Appointments

To Do
- ○
- ○
- ○
- ○
- ○
- ○

Cravings

Symptoms

General Health

Special Memories & Notes

"Dear Baby"

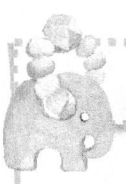

Love, Mom

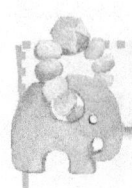

First Trimester — Week 11

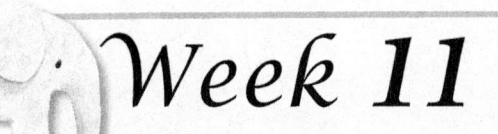

Baby's Development

Baby's Weight	
Baby's Size	_____ cm/in
Compares to a...	

About Me

Emotionally I am feeling

My Weight	
My Belly Size	

Events and Appointments	To Do		
	○	Cravings	
	○		
	○	Symptoms	
	○		
	○	General Health	
	○		

Special Memories & Notes

"Dear Baby"

Love, Mom

First Trimester

Week 12

Baby's Development

- Baby's Weight
- Baby's Size _____ cm/in
- Compares to a...

About Me

Emotionally I am feeling

- My Weight
- My Belly Size

Events and Appointments	To Do	
	○	Cravings
	○	
	○	Symptoms
	○	
	○	General Health
	○	

Special Memories & Notes

"Dear Baby"

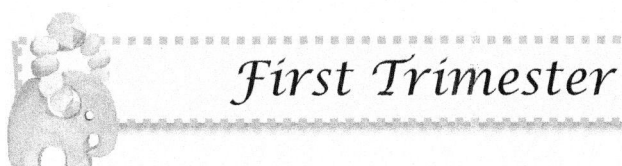

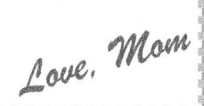

Love, Mom

Second Trimester

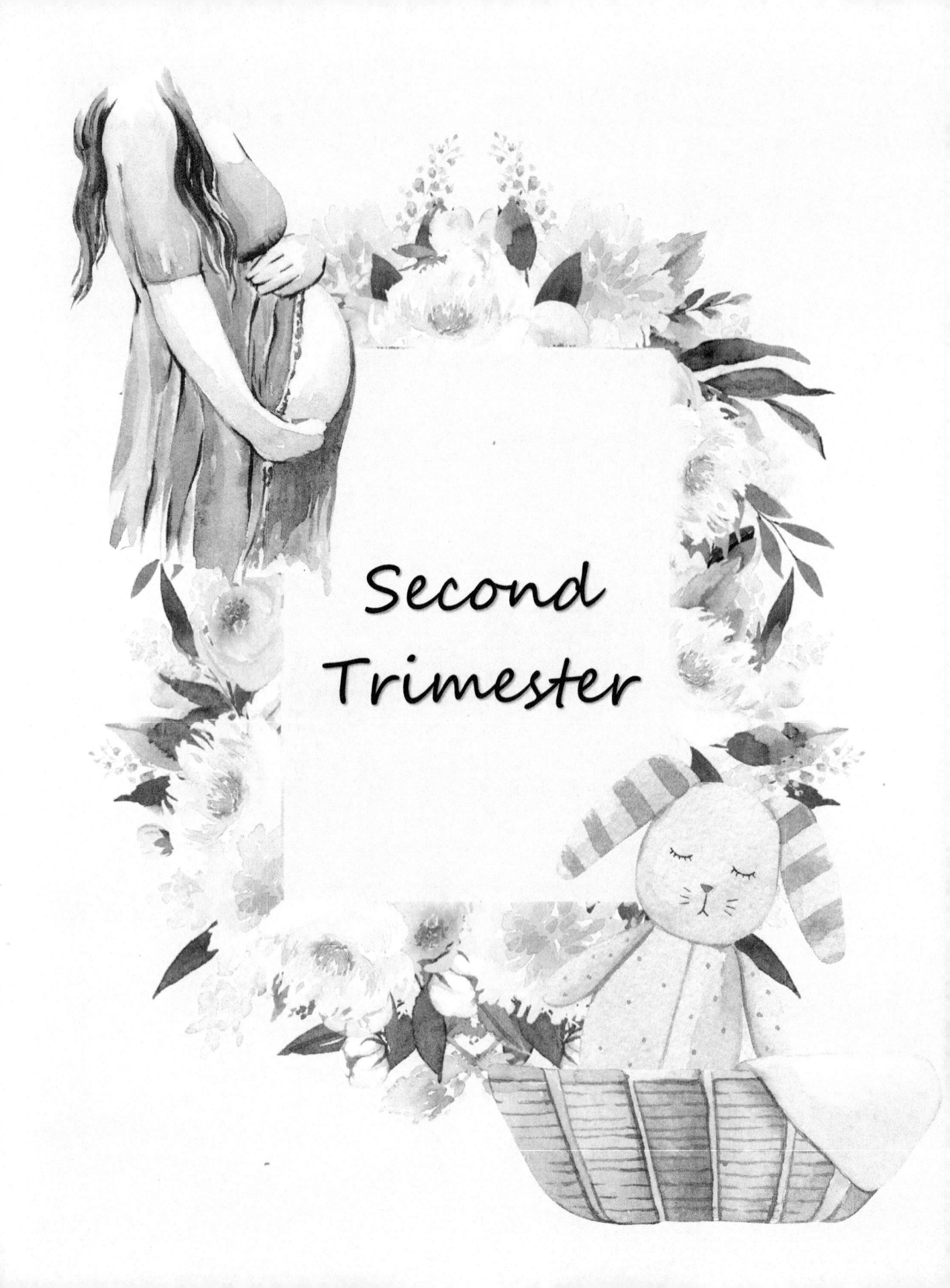

Second Trimester

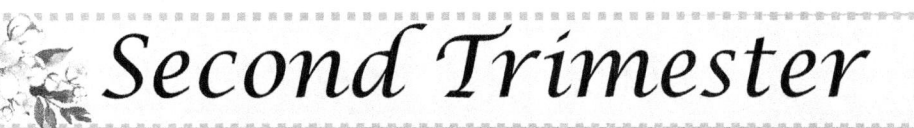

What to Expect

Notes

Preparation Checklist

- ○
- ○
- ○
- ○
- ○
- ○
- ○
- ○
- ○
- ○
- ○
- ○
- ○

I am excited for

I am anxious about

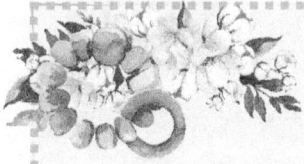

Second Trimester Checklist

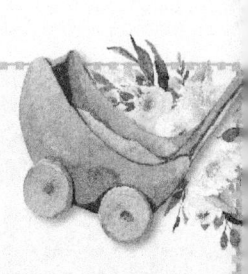

- ☐ Make pregnancy announcement
- ☐ Learn what to expect during prenatal visits
- ☐ Maintain healthy eating and exercise habits
- ☐ Decide if you want to find out baby's gender
- ☐ Start a baby registry
- ☐ Begin planning the nursery
- ☐ Do you want a baby shower? Who is the organizer?
- ☐ Announce your pregnancy to your employer
- ☐ Investigate childcare options
- ☐ Start short-listing baby names
- ☐ Shop for maternity wear
- ☐ Sign up for antenatal classes
- ☐ Focus on including your partner
- ☐ Start planning the nursery
- ☐ Continue taking weekly photos of your bump
- ☐ Begin a stretch mark prevention regime
- ☐ Make a dentist appointment
- ☐
- ☐
- ☐
- ☐
- ☐
- ☐

Notes

Second Trimester

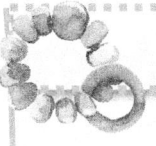

Week 13

Baby's Development

Baby's Weight	
Baby's Size	_____ cm/in
Compares to a...	

About Me

Emotionally I am feeling

My Weight	
My Belly Size	

Events and Appointments	To Do	
	○	Cravings
	○	
	○	Symptoms
	○	
	○	General Health
	○	

Special Memories & Notes

"Dear Baby"

Love, Mom

Second Trimester — Week 14

Baby's Development

- Baby's Weight
- Baby's Size _____ cm/in
- Compares to a...

About Me

Emotionally I am feeling

- My Weight
- My Belly Size

Events and Appointments	To Do	
	☐	Cravings
	☐	
	☐	Symptoms
	☐	
	☐	General Health
	☐	

Special Memories & Notes

"Dear Baby"

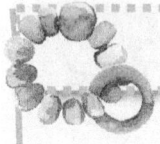

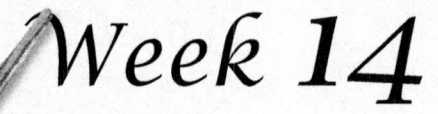

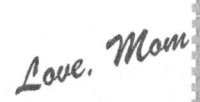

Love, Mom

Second Trimester

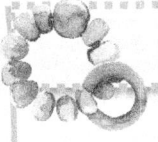

Week 15

Baby's Development

- Baby's Weight
- Baby's Size _____ cm/in
- Compares to a...

About Me

Emotionally I am feeling

- My Weight
- My Belly Size

Events and Appointments	To Do
	○
	○
	○
	○
	○
	○

Cravings

Symptoms

General Health

Special Memories & Notes

"Dear Baby"

Love, Mom

Second Trimester

Week 16

Baby's Development		Baby's Weight	
		Baby's Size	_____ cm/in
		Compares to a...	

About Me		My Weight	
Emotionally I am feeling		My Belly Size	

Events and Appointments	To Do		
	○	Cravings	
	○		
	○	Symptoms	
	○		
	○	General Health	
	○		

Special Memories & Notes

"Dear Baby"

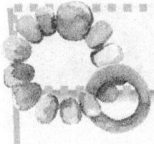

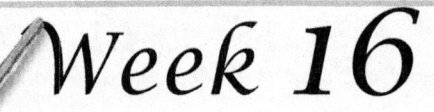

Love, Mom

Second Trimester — Week 17

Baby's Development

Baby's Weight	
Baby's Size	_____ cm/in
Compares to a…	

About Me

Emotionally I am feeling

My Weight	
My Belly Size	

Events and Appointments	To Do	
	○	Cravings
	○	
	○	Symptoms
	○	
	○	General Health
	○	

Special Memories & Notes

"Dear Baby"

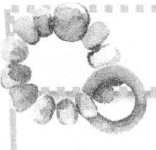

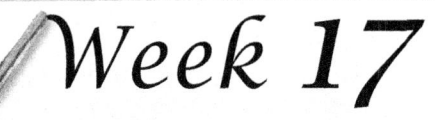

Love, Mom

Second Trimester

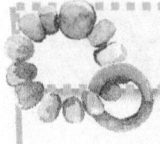

Week 18

Baby's Development

- Baby's Weight
- Baby's Size _____ cm/in
- Compares to a...

About Me
Emotionally I am feeling

- My Weight
- My Belly Size

Events and Appointments	To Do
	○
	○
	○
	○
	○
	○

Cravings

Symptoms

General Health

Special Memories & Notes

"Dear Baby"

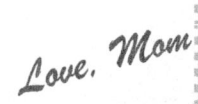

Love, Mom

Second Trimester
Week 19

Baby's Development

- Baby's Weight
- Baby's Size _____ cm/in
- Compares to a...

About Me

Emotionally I am feeling

- My Weight
- My Belly Size

Events and Appointments	To Do	
	○	Cravings
	○	
	○	Symptoms
	○	
	○	General Health
	○	

Special Memories & Notes

"Dear Baby"

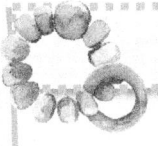

Love, Mom

Second Trimester

Week 20

Baby's Development

Baby's Weight	
Baby's Size	_____ cm/in
Compares to a...	

About Me

Emotionally I am feeling

My Weight	
My Belly Size	

Events and Appointments	To Do		
	○	Cravings	
	○		
	○	Symptoms	
	○		
	○	General Health	
	○		

Special Memories & Notes

"Dear Baby"

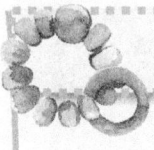

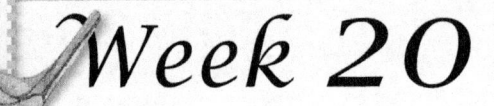

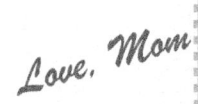

Love, Mom

Second Trimester

Week 21

Baby's Development

Baby's Weight	
Baby's Size	_____ cm/in
Compares to a...	

About Me

Emotionally I am feeling

My Weight	
My Belly Size	

Events and Appointments	To Do		
	○	Cravings	
	○		
	○	Symptoms	
	○		
	○	General Health	
	○		

Special Memories & Notes

"Dear Baby"

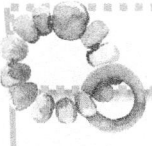

Love, Mom

Second Trimester
Week 22

Baby's Development

Baby's Weight

Baby's Size _____ cm/in

Compares to a...

About Me

Emotionally I am feeling

My Weight

My Belly Size

Events and Appointments	To Do	
	☐	Cravings
	☐	
	☐	Symptoms
	☐	
	☐	General Health
	☐	

Special Memories & Notes

"Dear Baby"

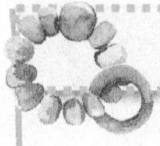

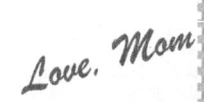

Love, Mom

Second Trimester

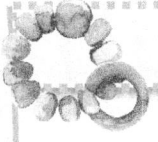

Week 23

Baby's Development

- Baby's Weight
- Baby's Size _____ cm/in
- Compares to a...

About Me
Emotionally I am feeling

- My Weight
- My Belly Size

Events and Appointments	To Do
	○
	○
	○
	○
	○
	○

Cravings

Symptoms

General Health

Special Memories & Notes

"Dear Baby"

Love, Mom

Second Trimester — Week 24

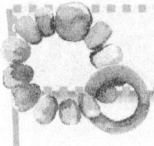

Baby's Development

Baby's Weight	
Baby's Size	_____ cm/in
Compares to a…	

About Me

Emotionally I am feeling

My Weight	
My Belly Size	

Events and Appointments	To Do		
	○	Cravings	
	○		
	○	Symptoms	
	○		
	○	General Health	
	○		

Special Memories & Notes

"Dear Baby"

Love, Mom

Second Trimester

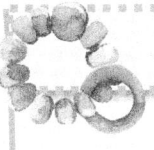

Week 25

Baby's Development

Baby's Weight	
Baby's Size	_____ cm/in
Compares to a...	

About Me

Emotionally I am feeling

My Weight	
My Belly Size	

Events and Appointments

To Do
- ○
- ○
- ○
- ○
- ○
- ○

Cravings

Symptoms

General Health

Special Memories & Notes

"Dear Baby"

Love, Mom

Second Trimester
Week 26

Baby's Development

Baby's Weight

Baby's Size _____ cm/in

Compares to a...

About Me

My Weight

Emotionally I am feeling

My Belly Size

Events and Appointments	To Do	
	○	Cravings
	○	
	○	Symptoms
	○	
	○	General Health
	○	

Special Memories & Notes

"Dear Baby"

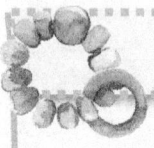

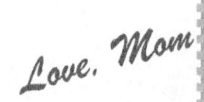

Love, Mom

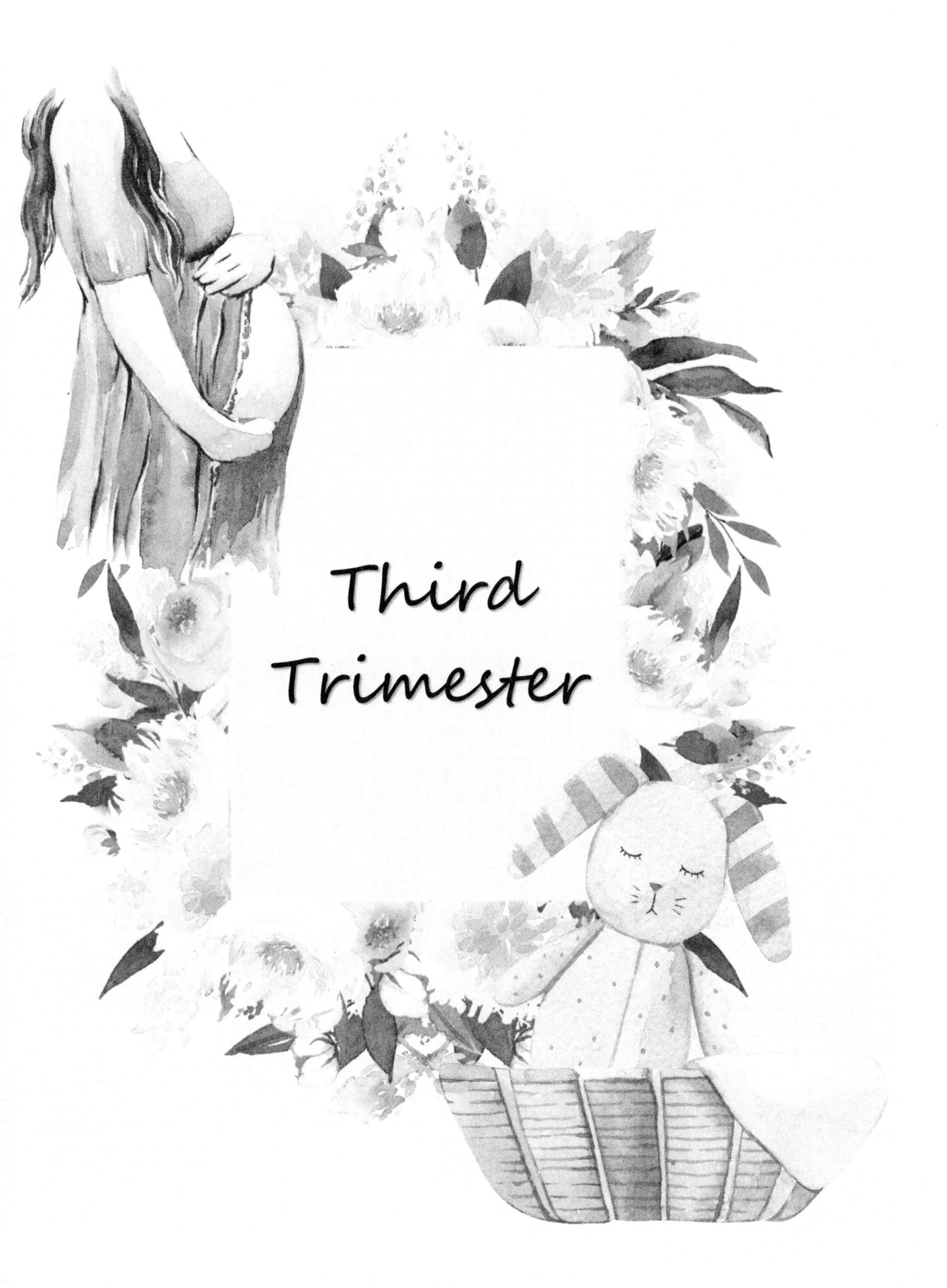

Third Trimester

Third Trimester

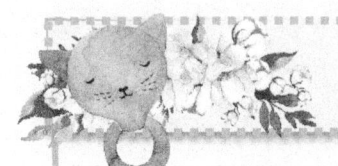

What to Expect

Preparation Checklist

- ○
- ○
- ○
- ○
- ○
- ○
- ○
- ○
- ○
- ○
- ○
- ○
- ○

Notes

I am excited for

I am anxious about

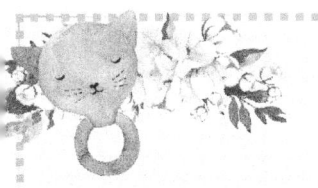

Third Trimester Checklist

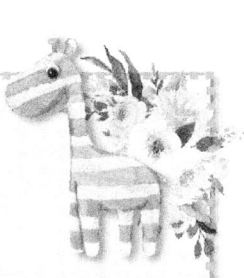

Task		Notes
Spring clean the house	○	
Organize hospital tour	○	
Pack hospital bags for you, baby and your partner	○	
Prepare your post-partum kit	○	
Stock up and sterilize all feeding equipment & supplies	○	
Study up on what to expect during labor	○	
Get baby car seat installed	○	
Finalize baby's name	○	
Ensure finances are in check for the next few months	○	
Spend quality time with other children	○	
Make final touches to nursery	○	
Wash all baby clothes and linens	○	
Finalize your preferred and alternate birth plan	○	
Prepare freezer meals	○	
	○	
	○	
	○	
	○	
	○	
	○	
	○	
	○	

Third Trimester

Week 27

Baby's Development

Baby's Weight

Baby's Size _____ cm/in

Compares to a...

About Me

My Weight

Emotionally I am feeling

My Belly Size

Events and Appointments	To Do	
	○	Cravings
	○	
	○	Symptoms
	○	
	○	General Health
	○	

Special Memories & Notes

"Dear Baby"

Love, Mom

Third Trimester

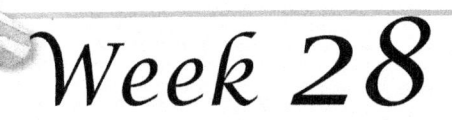

Week 28

Baby's Development

Baby's Weight

Baby's Size

Compares to a...

_____ cm/in

About Me

Emotionally I am feeling

My Weight

My Belly Size

Events and Appointments	To Do
	○
	○
	○
	○
	○
	○

Cravings

Symptoms

General Health

Special Memories & Notes

"Dear Baby"

Love, Mom

Third Trimester

Week 29

Baby's Development

Baby's Weight	
Baby's Size	_____ cm/in
Compares to a...	

About Me

Emotionally I am feeling

My Weight	
My Belly Size	

Events and Appointments	To Do		
	○	Cravings	
	○		
	○	Symptoms	
	○		
	○	General Health	
	○		

Special Memories & Notes

"Dear Baby"

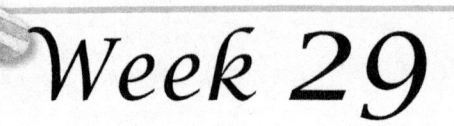

Love, Mom

Third Trimester

Week 30

Baby's Development

Baby's Weight	
Baby's Size	cm/in
Compares to a...	

About Me

Emotionally I am feeling

My Weight
My Belly Size

Events and Appointments	To Do		
	○	Cravings	
	○		
	○	Symptoms	
	○		
	○	General Health	
	○		

Special Memories & Notes

"Dear Baby"

Love, Mom

Third Trimester

Week 31

Baby's Development

Baby's Weight	
Baby's Size	_____ cm/in
Compares to a...	

About Me

Emotionally I am feeling

My Weight	
My Belly Size	

Events and Appointments	To Do	
	○	Cravings
	○	
	○	Symptoms
	○	
	○	General Health
	○	

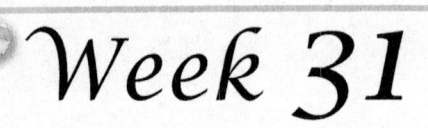

Special Memories & Notes

"Dear Baby"

Love, Mom

Third Trimester

Week 32

Baby's Development

- Baby's Weight
- Baby's Size
- _____ cm/in
- Compares to a…

About Me

Emotionally I am feeling

- My Weight
- My Belly Size

Events and Appointments

To Do
- ○
- ○
- ○
- ○
- ○
- ○

Cravings

Symptoms

General Health

Special Memories & Notes

"Dear Baby"

Love, Mom

Third Trimester

Week 33

Baby's Development

Baby's Weight	
Baby's Size	_____ cm/in
Compares to a...	

About Me

Emotionally I am feeling

My Weight	
My Belly Size	

Events and Appointments	To Do		
	○	Cravings	
	○		
	○	Symptoms	
	○		
	○	General Health	
	○		

Special Memories & Notes

"Dear Baby"

Love, Mom

Third Trimester

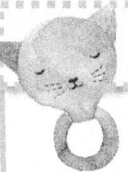

Week 34

Baby's Development

Baby's Weight	
Baby's Size	_____ cm/in
Compares to a...	

About Me

Emotionally I am feeling

My Weight	
My Belly Size	

Events and Appointments	To Do
	○
	○
	○
	○
	○
	○

Cravings

Symptoms

General Health

Special Memories & Notes

"Dear Baby"

Love, Mom

Third Trimester

Week 35

Baby's Development

- Baby's Weight
- Baby's Size
- Compares to a...

_____ cm/in

About Me

Emotionally I am feeling

- My Weight
- My Belly Size

Events and Appointments	To Do
	○
	○
	○
	○
	○
	○

Cravings

Symptoms

General Health

Special Memories & Notes

"Dear Baby"

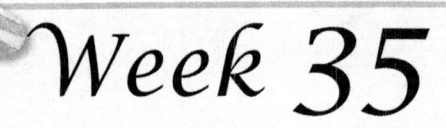

Love, Mom

Third Trimester

Week 36

Baby's Development

Baby's Weight

Baby's Size

_____ cm/in

Compares to a...

About Me

Emotionally I am feeling

My Weight

My Belly Size

Events and Appointments	To Do
	○
	○
	○
	○
	○
	○

Cravings

Symptoms

General Health

Special Memories & Notes

"Dear Baby"

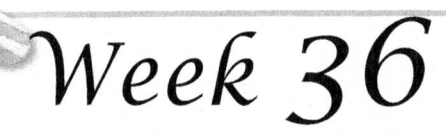

Love, Mom

Third Trimester

Week 37

Baby's Development

Baby's Weight	
Baby's Size	_____ cm/in
Compares to a...	

About Me
Emotionally I am feeling

My Weight	
My Belly Size	

Events and Appointments	To Do	
	○	Cravings
	○	
	○	Symptoms
	○	
	○	General Health
	○	

Special Memories & Notes

"Dear Baby"

Love, Mom

Third Trimester

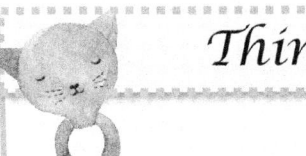

Week 38

Baby's Development

Baby's Weight	
Baby's Size	_____ cm/in
Compares to a...	

About Me

Emotionally I am feeling

My Weight	
My Belly Size	

Events and Appointments

To Do
-
-
-
-
-
-

Cravings

Symptoms

General Health

Special Memories & Notes

"Dear Baby"

Love, Mom

Third Trimester
Week 39

Baby's Development

- Baby's Weight
- Baby's Size _____ cm/in
- Compares to a...

About Me
Emotionally I am feeling

- My Weight
- My Belly Size

Events and Appointments	To Do	
	○	Cravings
	○	
	○	Symptoms
	○	
	○	General Health
	○	

Special Memories & Notes

"Dear Baby"

Love, Mom

Third Trimester

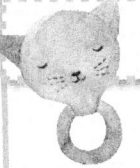

Week 40

Baby's Development

- Baby's Weight
- Baby's Size
- Compares to a...

cm/in

About Me

Emotionally I am feeling

- My Weight
- My Belly Size

Events and Appointments	To Do
	○
	○
	○
	○
	○
	○

Cravings

Symptoms

General Health

Special Memories & Notes

"Dear Baby"

Love, Mom

You've Arrived!

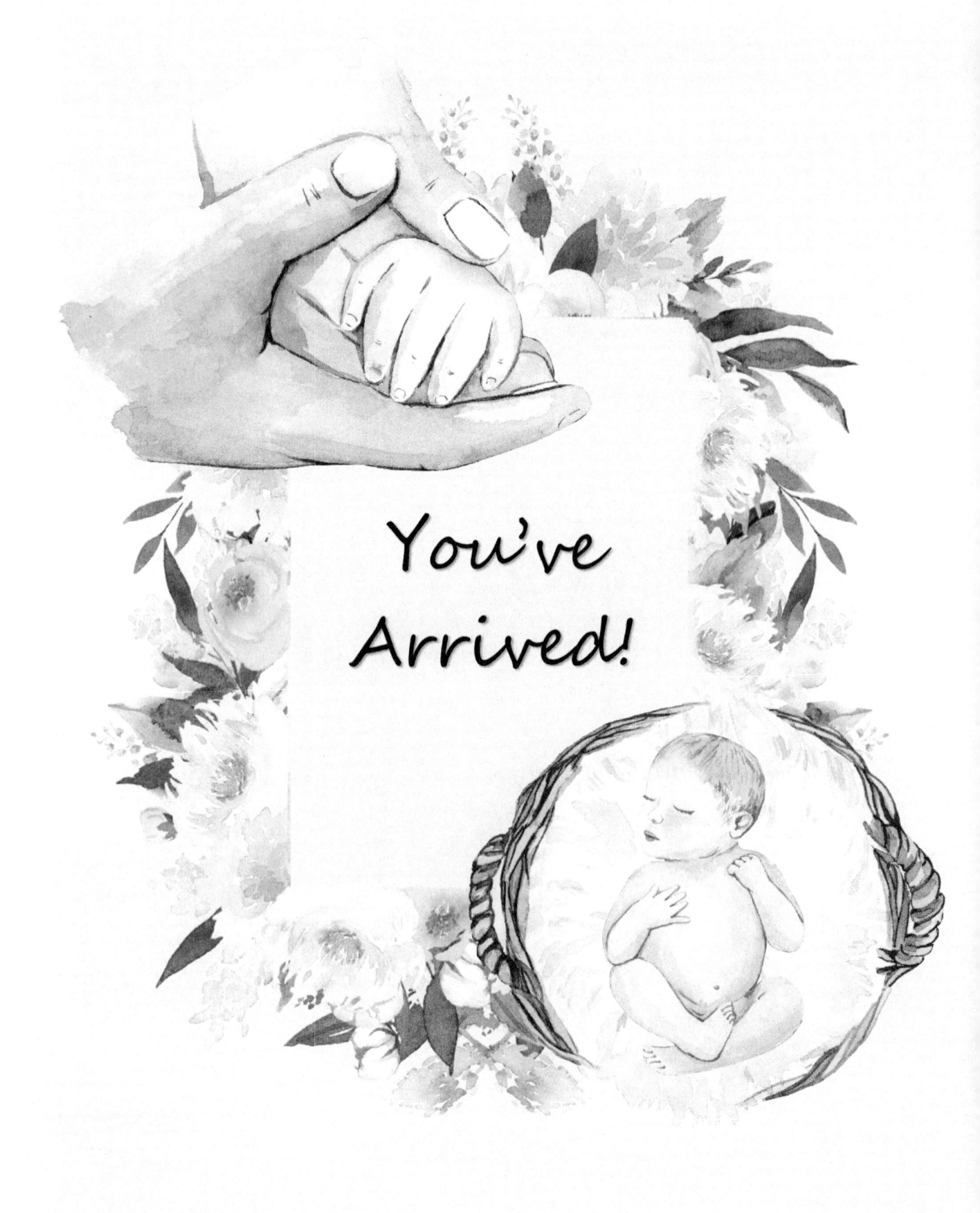

Welcome!

Full names _____

Date _____ Time _____ Weight _____

Who was there_____

When I went into labor

My labor and birthing experience

How I felt when I first saw you

How your father reacted when he first saw you

The first thing you did

How we announced to the world

My special note to you, as we start this new journey together

Love, Mommy

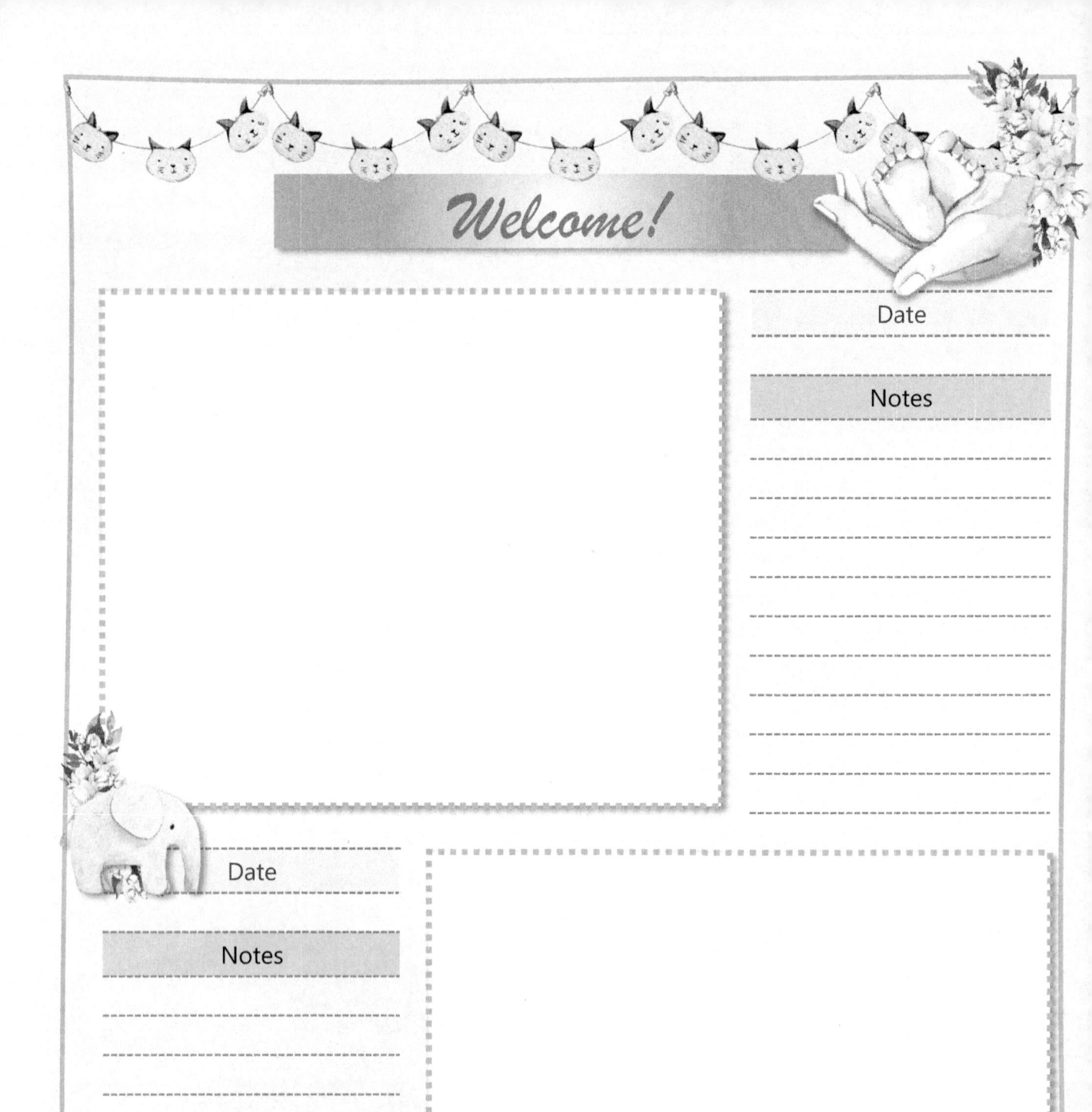

Welcome!

Date

Notes

Date

Notes

Month 1

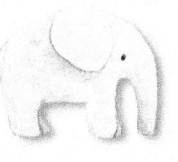

From _____ **to** _____

Appointments and Outings

	Date	Time	Preparation	Notes
My checkups				
Baby's checkups				
Mother & Baby Group				
Inoculations				

To Do

- ○
- ○
- ○
- ○
- ○
- ○
- ○
- ○
- ○
- ○
- ○
- ○
- ○
- ○
- ○

I'm excited for

Notes

Month 1 Milestones

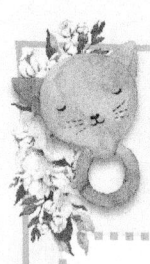

Date

Weight

Length

Baby Firsts

Special Memories

Month 2

From _____ **to** _____

Appointments and Outings

	Date	Time	Preparation	Notes
My checkups				
Baby's checkups				
Mother & Baby Group				
Inoculations				

To Do
- ○
- ○
- ○
- ○
- ○
- ○
- ○
- ○
- ○
- ○
- ○
- ○
- ○
- ○
- ○

I'm excited for

Notes

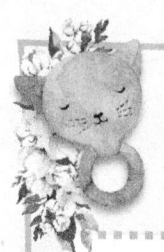

Month 2 Milestones

Date

Weight

Length

Baby Firsts

Special Memories

Month 3

From _____ **to** _____

Appointments and Outings

	Date	Time	Preparation	Notes
My checkups				
Baby's checkups				
Mother & Baby Group				
Inoculations				

To Do

- ○ _____
- ○ _____
- ○ _____
- ○ _____
- ○ _____
- ○ _____
- ○ _____
- ○ _____
- ○ _____
- ○ _____
- ○ _____
- ○ _____
- ○ _____
- ○ _____
- ○ _____

I'm excited for

Notes

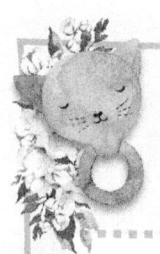

Month 3 Milestones

Date

Weight

Length

Baby Firsts

Special Memories

Month 4

From _____ **to** _____

Appointments and Outings

	Date	Time	Preparation	Notes
My checkups				
Baby's checkups				
Mother & Baby Group				
Inoculations				

To Do

- ○
- ○
- ○
- ○
- ○
- ○
- ○
- ○
- ○
- ○
- ○
- ○
- ○
- ○
- ○

I'm excited for

Notes

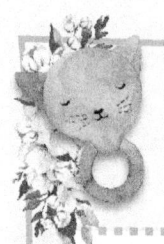

Month 4 Milestones

Date

Weight

Length

Baby Firsts

Special Memories

Month 5

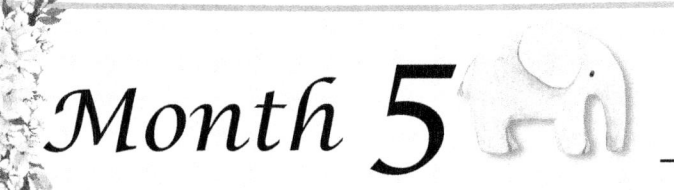

From _____ to _____

Appointments and Outings

	Date	Time	Preparation	Notes
My checkups				
Baby's checkups				
Mother & Baby Group				
Inoculations				

To Do

- ○
- ○
- ○
- ○
- ○
- ○
- ○
- ○
- ○
- ○
- ○
- ○
- ○
- ○
- ○

I'm excited for

Notes

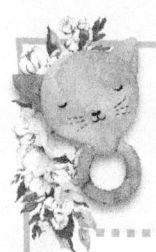

Month 5 Milestones

Date

Weight

Length

Baby Firsts

Special Memories

Month 6

From _____ **to** _____

Appointments and Outings

	Date	Time	Preparation	Notes
My checkups				
Baby's checkups				
Mother & Baby Group				
Inoculations				

To Do
- ○
- ○
- ○
- ○
- ○
- ○
- ○
- ○
- ○
- ○
- ○
- ○
- ○
- ○
- ○
- ○

I'm excited for

Notes

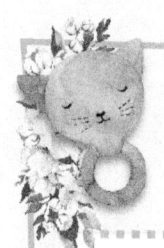

Month 6 Milestones

Date

Weight

Length

Baby Firsts

Special Memories

Journaling

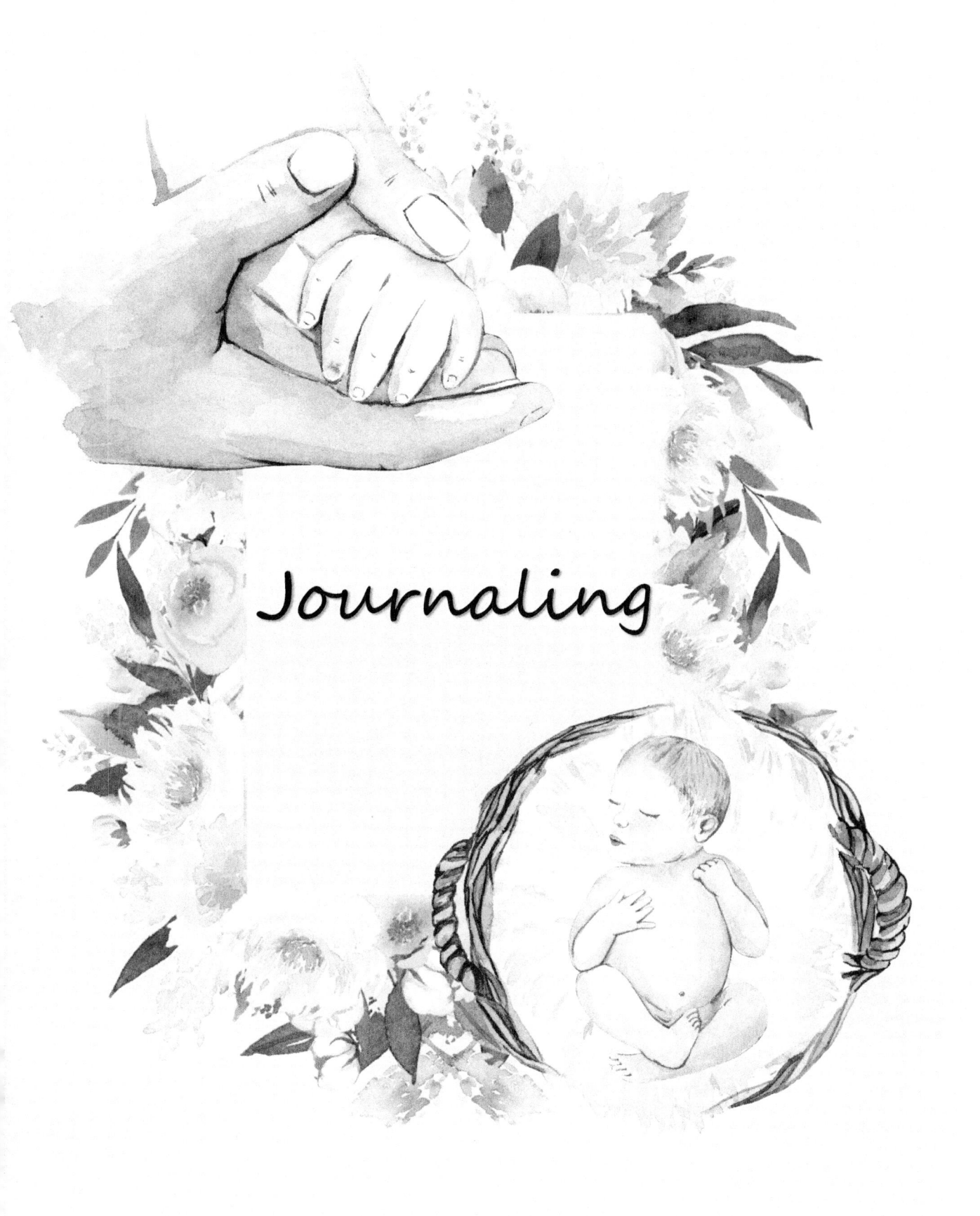

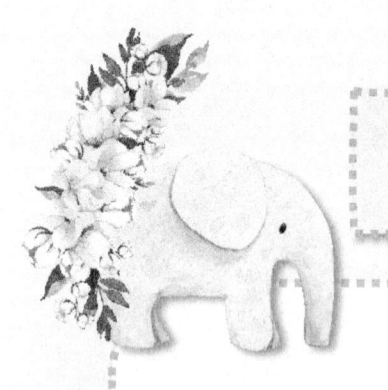

"Dear Baby"

___ / ___ / ___

Love, Mom

"Dear Baby"

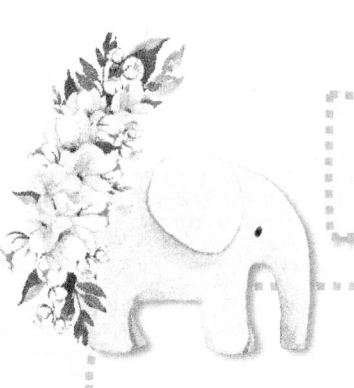

___ / ___ / ___

Love, Mom

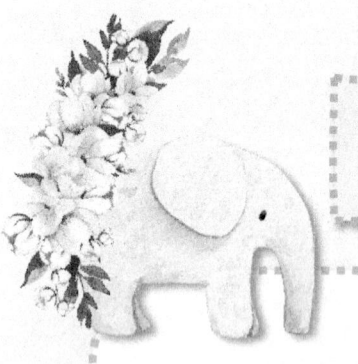

"Dear Baby"

___ / ___ / ___

Love, Mom

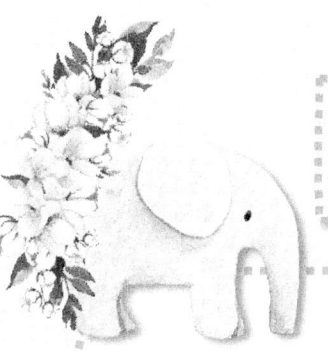

"Dear Baby"

___ / ___ / ___

Love, Mom

"Dear Baby"

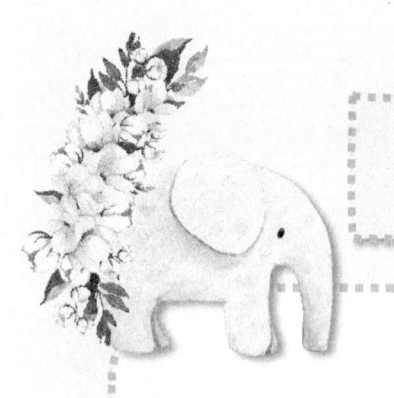

___ / ___ / ___

Love, Mom

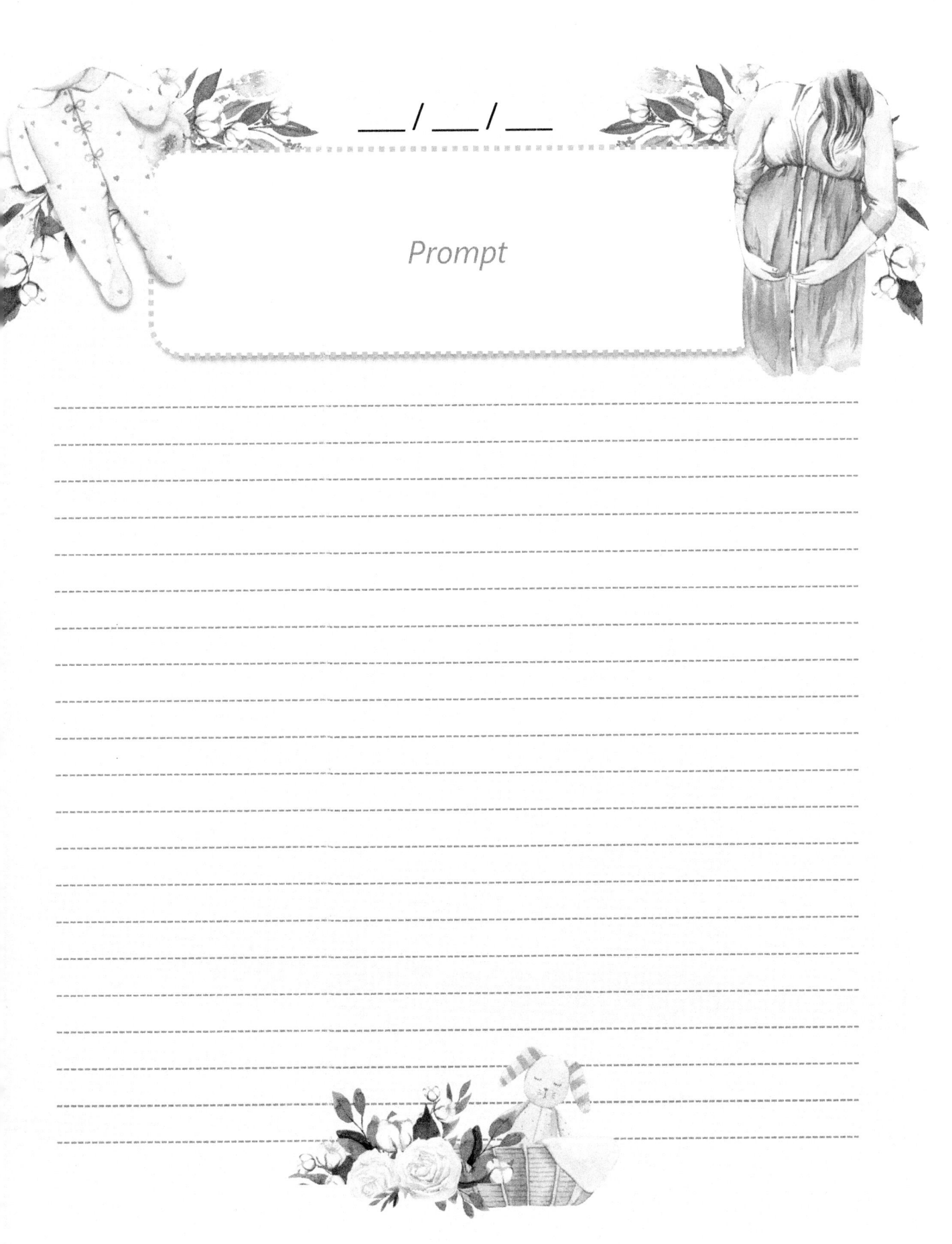

___/___/___

Prompt

___/___/___

Printed in Great Britain
by Amazon